PREGNANCY AND
RENAL DISORDERS

Other titles in the *New Clinical Applications* Series:

Dermatology (Series Editor Dr J. L. Verbov)
Dermatological Surgery
Superficial Fungal Infections
Talking Points in Dermatology – I
Treatment in Dermatology
Current Concepts in Contact Dermatitis
Talking Points in Dermatology – II
Tumours, Lymphomas and Selected Paraproteinaemias
Relationships in Dermatology

Cardiology (Series Editor Dr D. Longmore)
Cardiology Screening

Rheumatology (Series Editors Dr J. J. Calabro and Dr W. Carson Dick)
Ankylosing Spondylitis
Infections and Arthritis

Nephrology (Series Editor Professor G. R. D. Catto)
Continuous Ambulatory Peritoneal Dialysis
Management of Renal Hypertension
Chronic Renal Failure
Calculus Disease
Pregnancy and Renal Disorders
Multisystem Diseases
Glomerulonephritis I
Glomerulonephritis II

NEW
CLINICAL
APPLICATIONS
NEPHROLOGY

PREGNANCY AND RENAL DISORDERS

Editor

G. R. D. CATTO

DSc, MD, FRCP, (Lond., Edin. and Glasg.)

Professor in Medicine and Therapeutics
University of Aberdeen
UK

KLUWER ACADEMIC PUBLISHERS
DORDRECHT / BOSTON / LONDON

Distributors

for the United States and Canada: Kluwer Academic Publishers, PO Box 358, Accord Station, Hingham, MA 02018-0358, USA
for all other countries: Kluwer Academic Publishers Group, Distribution Center, PO Box 322, 3300 AH Dordrecht, The Netherlands

British Library Cataloguing in Publication Data

Pregnancy and renal disorders.
1. Pregnant women. Kidneys. Diseases
I. Catto, Graeme R.D. (Graeme Robertson Dawson), *1945–* II. Series
618.3'26

Library of Congress Cataloging-in-Publication Data

Pregnancy and renal disorders/editor, G.R.D. Catto.
p. cm.—(New clinical applications. Nephrology)
Includes bibliographies and index.

ISBN-13: 978-94-010-7680-7 e-ISBN-13: 978-94-009-2615-8

DOI: 10.1007/978-94-009-2615-8

1. Kidney diseases in pregnancy. I. Catto, Graeme R. D.
II. Series.
[DNLM: 1. Kidney Diseases—in pregnancy. 2. Pregnancy Complications. WJ 300 P923]
RG580.K5P74 1988
618.3'26—dc19
DNLM/DLC
for Library of Congress 88-8369
CIP

Published in the United Kingdom by Kluwer Academic Publishers, PO Box 55, Lancaster, UK.

Kluwer Academic Publishers BV incorporates the publishing programmes of D. Reidel, Martinus Nijhoff, Dr W. Junk and MTP Press.

Butler & Tanner Ltd, Frome and London

CONTENTS

LIST OF AUTHORS

H. A. Lee
Department of Renal Medicine
University of Southampton
St Mary's Hospital
Portsmouth
Hampshire PO3 6AD
UK

A. M. MacLeod
Department of Medicine and Therapeutics
University of Aberdeen
Polwarth Building
Foresterhill
Aberdeen AB9 2ZD
UK

D. W. M. Pearson
Diabetic Clinic
Woolmanhill
Aberdeen Royal Infirmary
Aberdeen AB9 1GS
UK

H. W. Sutherland
Department of Obstetrics and Gynaecology
Aberdeen Maternity Hospital
Cornhill Road
Aberdeen AB9 2ZA
UK

C. P. Swainson
Medical Renal Unit
Department of Medicine
Royal Infirmary
Edinburgh EH3 9YW
UK

K. Verrier Jones
Department of Child Health
University of Wales College of Medicine
Royal Infirmary
Cardiff CF2 1SZ
UK

SERIES EDITOR'S FOREWORD

Almost every practising doctor will admit to difficulty in knowing how best to investigate, treat and advise the pregnant patient with renal problems. These doubts and difficulties may be exacerbated if the patient seeks pre-pregnancy advice – would a possible pregnancy cause a deterioration in renal function, what are the risks of the pregnancy for mother and baby? As the general public become more informed on medical matters these questions are being asked more frequently and doctors must be prepared to offer advice which is based on detailed factual knowledge.

This book examines some of these increasingly common clinical problems. Each chapter has been written by a recognized expert in the field and provides the type of specific information now expected by discerning patients. The advances in treatment of the last decade clearly indicate that a knowledge of pregnancy and renal disorders is essential for doctors in many branches of medical practice.

G. R.D. Catto

ABOUT THE EDITOR

Dr Graeme R. D. Catto is Professor in Medicine and Therapeutics at the University of Aberdeen and Honorary Consultant Physician/Nephrologist to the Grampian Health Board. His current interest in transplant immunology was stimulated as a Harkness Fellow at Harvard Medical School and the Peter Bent Brighton Hospital, Boston, USA. He is a member of many medical societies including the Association of Physicians of Great Britain and Ireland, the Renal Association and the Transplantation Society. He has published widely on transplant and reproductive immunology, calcium metabolism and general nephrology.

1

URINARY TRACT INFECTION

K. VERRIER JONES

INTRODUCTION

It is well known that symptomatic urinary tract infection, particularly acute pyelonephritis, occurs more often during pregnancy than in non-pregnant women of comparable age or younger or older women. However, there is no evidence that asymptomatic bacteriuria (ASB) is more common during pregnancy than in non-pregnant women[1]. Because of the severe acute illness often produced during pregnancy as a result of urinary tract infection, and because this may have an adverse effect on the course of the pregnancy and on the fetus, there has been considerable interest in this condition. In the pre-antibiotic era it was possible to observe the natural history of acute pyelonephritis[2,3]. Some unfortunate women continued to have fever and loin pain for many weeks. In some, symptoms improved after delivery, whilst in others, symptoms continued into the puerperium. In 1939, Weiss and Parker vividly described the course of a woman with chronic pyelonephritis, with pregnancy-associated hypertension and toxaemia, who subsequently developed dysuria, backache, retinal haemorrhages, acute pyelonephritis, septicaemia and anaemia in relation to one successful pregnancy and one which ended in a spontaneous abortion at 19 weeks[4]. Whilst this type of illness with severe underlying renal disease is seen only occasionally, and both hypertension and infection can be treated successfully, acute pyelonephritis remains a serious, occasionally life threatening, but treatable condition in pregnancy. The incidence and morbidity of acute pyelonephritis and its complications can be significantly reduced by screening for ASB[5] and by prompt diagnosis and early treatment of any cases of symptomatic infections when they occur.

There are many different clinical presentations of urinary tract infection and those which are relevant to pregnancy will be discussed in further detail later in this chapter. Urinary infection in women is frequently a persisting or recurring condition[6]. The relationship between covert infection, symptomatic infection, treatment and complications is summarised in Figure 1.1. There is little evidence that acute infection at the time of pregnancy causes permanent renal damage but transient abnormalities of renal function are present with upper urinary tract infection[7,8]. Acute renal failure is a rare complication of acute pyelonephritis in pregnancy but women with chronic pyelonephritis and impaired renal function may experience a more rapid decline in renal function following pregnancy[9], particularly if blood pressure is poorly controlled. Septicaemia and persisting or relapsing infection are usually confined to those women who have

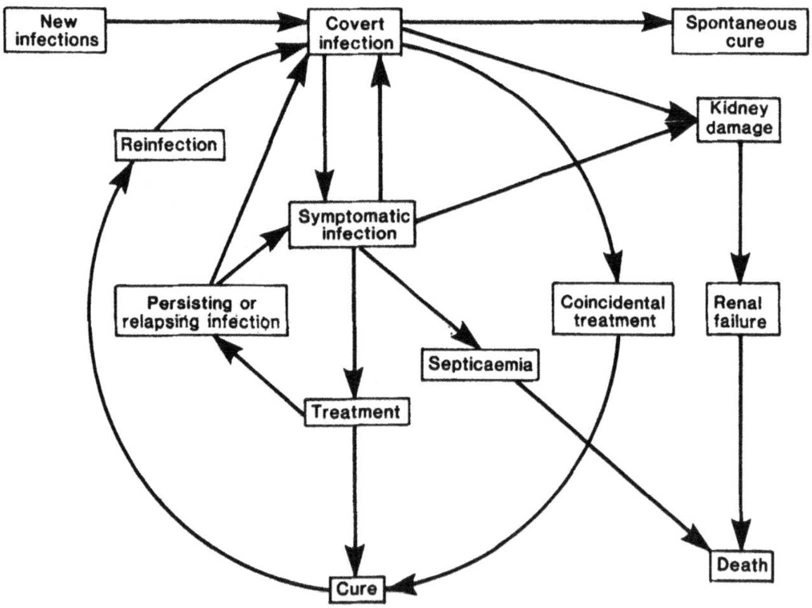

FIGURE 1.1 Relationship between asymptomatic and symptomatic infection, treatment, reinfection and renal damage

renal calculi or obstruction underlying acute pyelonephritis. Reinfection via the urethra following successful treatment is common in women prone to asymptomatic bacteriuria or recurrent symptomatic infection. Catheterization is an important iatrogenic cause of urinary infection in obstetric practice[10].

The aim of pregnancy is to produce a healthy infant. This complex process is readily upset. Any treatment must take into account the needs and well being of the infant who is significantly more vulnerable than the mother. The benefits of any treatment used to control urinary infection in the mother must be carefully balanced against the benefits and disadvantages of persisting maternal ill health and drug exposure to the infant in both the short and long term. These problems will be discussed in this chapter in the light of the altered host–parasite relationship which occurs in pregnancy.

PATHOGENESIS

Reservoir of organisms and route of entry

The vast majority of bacterial infections of the urinary tract are acquired as a result of ascending infection, although the evidence for this is largely circumstantial. The large bowel acts as a reservoir for organisms invading the urinary tract[11]. Those organisms, such as *Escherichia coli*, which commonly colonize the urinary tract have virulence factors which enable them to colonize the perineum, ascend the urethra and adhere and multiply in the lower and upper urinary tract[12]. *Bacteroides spp.*, which outnumber coliform organisms in the gut, rarely cause urinary tract infection unless there is a direct communication between the gut and the bladder. In women prone to recurrent urinary tract infection, Stamey and Sexton showed that periurethral colonization occurs prior to the development of bacteriuria[13] and that these women have lower levels of secretory IgA in the vagina than women not prone to urinary infection[14]. There is evidence that sexual intercourse increases the risk of bacterial entry into the urinary tract[15] and iatrogenic ascending infection may occur following catheterization[16].

Colonization of the bladder and bacterial growth in urine

The ability of bacteria to ascend the urethra, colonize the bladder and survive in the urinary tract depends on the host–parasite relationship. There is a fine balance between those host factors which favour bacterial growth and survival and those which work to eliminate bacteria. This relationship is subtly altered in pregnancy[17], and, although the prevalence of bacteriuria is not significantly different in women in the pregnant and non-pregnant states, the clinical manifestations may be significantly altered so that pregnant women are many times more likely than non-pregnant women to develop the symptoms and signs of acute pyelonephritis.

Bacteria adhere to the periurethral cells[13] and ascend the urethra. In the bladder, some organisms are free within the urine whilst others adhere to the urothelial cells and mucoid slime layer[18]. They are able to multiply using the small amount of glucose normally present in the urine as a source of energy[19]. Bacteria have shown a remarkable ability to survive and multiply in the variable conditions of pH and osmolality present in the urine, although bacterial growth is inhibited at the extremes of pH achieved in human urine[20]. The growth rate for *Escherichia coli* is reduced significantly in highly concentrated urine, particularly at low pH. A survey in South Wales showed that early morning urine samples from women were likely to have conditions of pH and osmolality which favour bacterial growth significantly more often than men, and urine obtained from pregnant women is usually suitable for bacterial growth[21]. Secretory IgA is present in normal urine but reduced in women prone to urinary tract infections[22].

Elimination of bacteria

Bacteria present in the bladder urine are normally eliminated during micturition[23] so that only those bacteria adherent to the wall of the bladder persist. The presence of a post-micturition residue allows a pool of infected urine to remain and may permit infection with organisms which would normally be eliminated. Multiplication of these remaining bacteria may perpetuate the infection[24]. In pregnancy, micturition patterns are altered, the bladder is compressed by the gravid uterus and the upper urinary tract, particularly the right kidney, is often dilated. This may also interfere with the normal mechanisms for bacterial elimination and thus predispose to infection. The presence of any underlying urological abnormality will also predispose to infection if urinary stasis or obstruction is present. The appearance of a dilated ureter and renal pelvis is common in pregnancy and may be expected to resolve during the months following delivery[25,26].

Mechanisms of inflammation and antibody response

Adherent bacteria in contact with the bladder wall cause inflammation by triggering the respiratory burst of polymorphonuclear leucocytes which in turn liberate chemical mediators of inflammation[27]. Simultaneously, the bacteria are attacked and destroyed by host defences. In some cases, bacterial adherence is mediated through fimbriae (Figure 1.2). Mannose sensitive fimbriae have been shown to be hydrophobic and capable of triggering the respiratory burst[28] whilst some mannose-resistant (p) fimbriae adhere to the globoside receptor present on cells of the urothelium[29]. There is evidence that the number of receptors expressed is under hormonal influence and may therefore be influenced by pregnancy[30]. The antibody response is influenced by the age of the patient, the site of infection, previous exposure to similar organisms and by the virulence characteristics of the invading organism[31]. Several workers have shown a relationship between acute pyelonephritis and the development of antibodies to the 'O' antigen of *Escherichia coli*[32–34]. In addition, there is evidence of antibody production in the bladder wall in response to infection but little evidence that these antibodies are important in preventing infection. Immunoglobulins present in the urine may also be important[35]. Thomas, Shelokov and Forland showed that organisms were often coated with antibody and that this phenomenon correlated with upper tract infection[36].

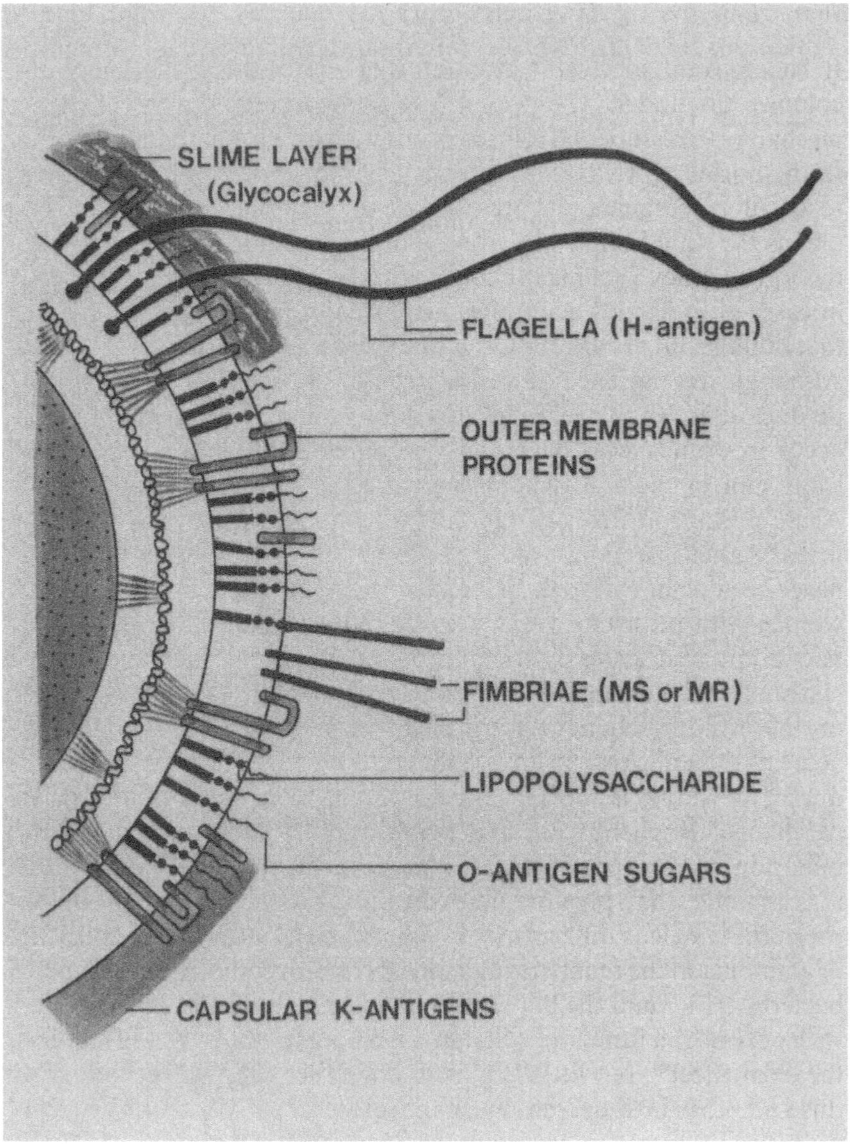

FIGURE 1.2 Schematic representation of cell wall of *Escherichia coli* showing the antigenic proteins which are responsible for the organism's virulence characteristics

Pathogenesis of acute pyelonephritis

If bacteria are successful in colonizing the bladder, they may also colonize the ureter. The presence of dilated ureters, whether due to mechanical pressure and altered urodynamics during pregnancy[37,38] or to the hormonal relaxation of collagen and smooth muscle, believed to occur in pregnancy[39], predisposes to bacterial colonization. Not only is the right kidney more prone to dilation during pregnancy, but the right kidney is clinically affected more often than the left kidney in cases of unilateral acute pyelonephritis of pregnancy[40], suggesting that dilatation of the ureter is an important predisposing factor. Although the presence of vesicoureteric reflux has been thought to predispose to acute pyelonephritis in pregnancy, these symptoms can occur in women who have had vesicoureteric reflux corrected surgically and in those in whom spontaneous resolution has occurred. Acute pyelonephritis is common in all women with a past history of urinary tract infection, even those in whom vesicoureteric reflux has never been demonstrated. In a recent study, El Katib *et al.* found that women with persisting vesicoureteric reflux had an increased risk of bacteriuria and acute pyelonephritis but this small increase was not statistically significant[41]. The presence of p fimbriae and the K antigen on the invading bacteria are thought to predispose to symptoms of acute pyelonephritis outside pregnancy but their role in pyelonephritis during pregnancy is unclear. *Escherichia coli* has a remarkable capacity to change its phenotypic expression and to undergo spontaneous mutation when exposed to different experimental conditions so that it is possible that phenotypic expression by *Escherichia coli* in the pregnant female is different from other clinical settings. The presence of ammonia in the renal medulla interferes with complement-mediated bacterial lysis[42] and the hyperosmolar conditions in this area interfere with polymorph function[43]. Serum has a natural ability to kill bacteria, the cidal effect[44], but little is known about the effect of pregnancy on this and other host defence mechanisms.

ASYMPTOMATIC BACTERIURIA

ASB is a common condition in females of all ages, approximately 1 in 20 women being affected, and there is no evidence to suggest that pregnancy affects the prevalence of this condition. Although the term 'asymptomatic' is used to describe these women who may remain bacteriuric for long periods of time and possibly throughout life, symptoms can often be elicited on careful questioning. Common symptoms include frequency, nocturia, suprapubic pain, dysuria, loin pain, backache and constipation[45]. The symptoms are often mild and have been present for a long time, so that they may be accepted as normal by that individual. There is, presumably, a symbiosis between the host and the parasite[46] which may continue for many years provided that the delicate balance is not disturbed. During pregnancy, this balance is changed and, in some women, acute pyelonephritis will develop with the same organism that has previously been responsible for asymptomatic infection. On the other hand, bacteriuria may resolve spontaneously at any time or as a result of coincidental treatment. During the short time course of pregnancy, ASB resolves spontaneously in approximately one third[47].

Concept of the colony count

The maximum concentration of organisms that urine can support is in the region of 10^7–10^8 per ml. Shortage of glucose and other nutrients probably prevents further bacterial multiplication so that the number of new organisms is balanced against the number dying. In the human bladder urine, this concentration of organisms may be present but the concentration of organisms may be reduced by frequent bladder emptying and unfavourable conditions for bacterial multiplication in the urine. Each live organism is capable of forming a colony and this phenomenon was utilized by Miles and Misra who first developed techniques for estimation of the colony count[48]. Kass[5,49] used the colony count to differentiate between bacteria found in the urine as a result of contamination and true bladder bacteriuria. Using bacterial colony counts on mid-stream urine samples, he showed that women with asymptomatic bacteriuria usually had a pure growth of organisms with counts of > 100 000 cfu/ml. Although a minority of women with ASB had lower colony counts, these low counts were more likely to occur as a result of contamination than with true bacteriuria (Figure 1.3), particularly if there was a mixed growth of organisms. His results showed that, if two urine samples show 'significant bacteriuria', there is a 96% chance that bacteriuria is present.

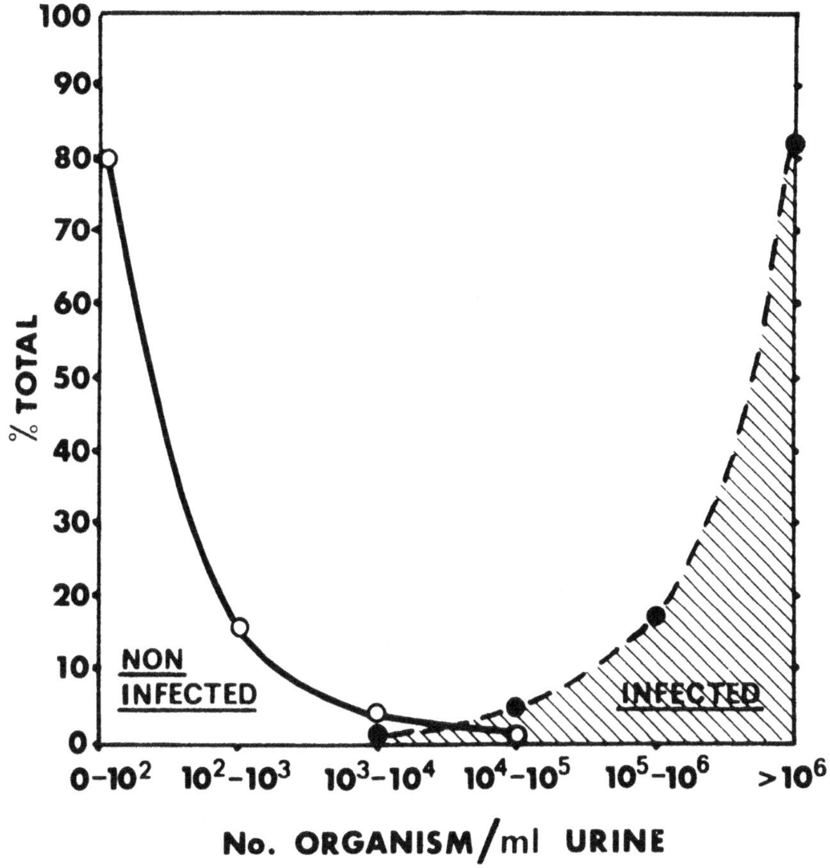

FIGURE 1.3 Bacterial colony counts obtained from women with infected and non-infected urine

Method of collection and transport to laboratory

There is a strong possibility that small numbers of organisms from the perineum or pubic hair may contaminate the sample. Many women have great difficulty in producing urine samples under the strict conditions of a conventionally collected mid-stream sample. In particular, they have difficulty in separating the labia adequately and in catching only the mid part of the urinary stream. It is difficult for a pregnant woman to hold the receiver and manipulate it in the toilet without putting her fingers in it. Thus true mid-stream samples are probably only obtained when the collection is closely supervised. If the perineum is cleansed, only green soap or water should be used. If an antiseptic solution is used there is a possibility that a small drip might enter the urine. This could prevent bacterial growth and thus mask an infection, particularly if reliance is placed on the colony count rather than microscopy, as is the case in most laboratories responsible for screening procedures.

It is essential that the urine is plated on culture media within two hours of collection. Delay in culturing the urine will lead to confusing results because of bacterial multiplication of contaminating organisms. This problem is significantly reduced if samples are stored at 4°C or if boric acid is added[50] since bacterial growth is inhibited under these conditions. Alternatively, the clinician can plate the urine immediately on to commercially prepared dipslides (Figure 1.4a) which can be transported to the laboratory or office for incubation at leisure[51]. The colony count can be interpreted without special training by comparison with a chart (Figure 1.4b). The nature and sensitivity of the infecting organism can be identified subsequently by subculture using conventional techniques[52]. Urine collected by suprapubic puncture will not be contaminated if the technique has been carried out correctly[53] but there is a small theoretical risk of contamination as a result of penetration of the rectum or vagina. Urethral catheterization also produces reliable urine samples with only a small risk of contamination. However, both these procedures are too invasive for routine use and catheterization has the added disadvantage that organisms may be introduced at the time the catheter is passed[10].

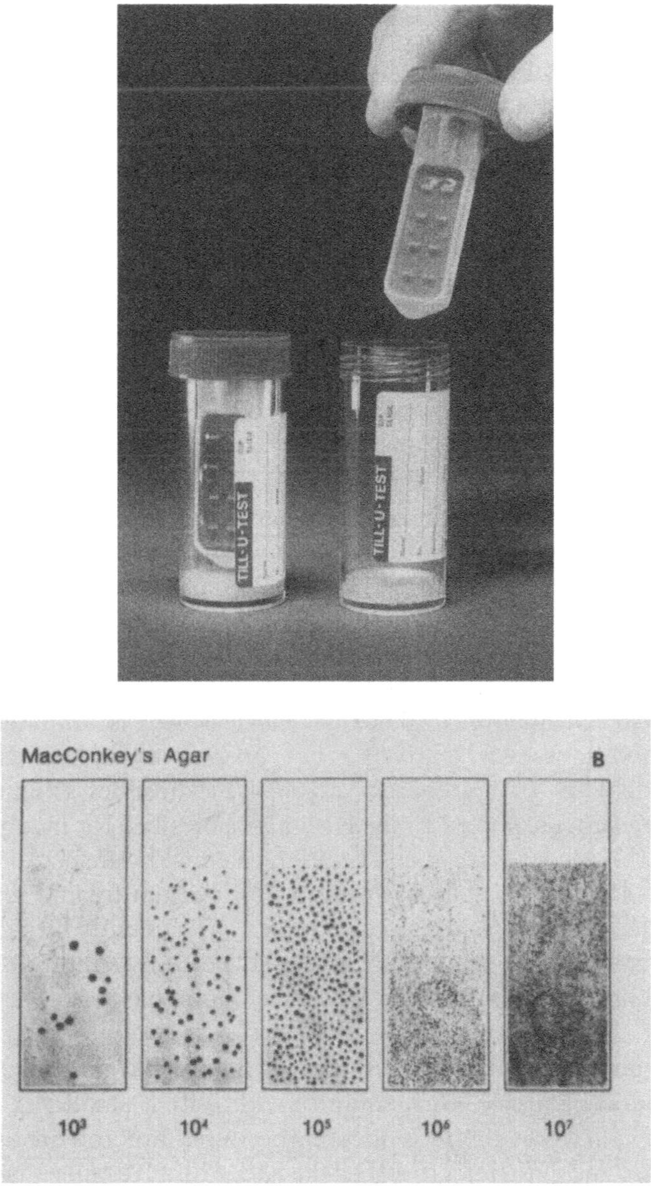

FIGURE 1.4 (a) Commercially prepared dipslides. (b) Appearance of dipslide after 24–72 h incubation. Colony count can be assessed by comparison with charts shown above

Screening methods

The original techniques for counting viable organisms or colonies in solid media were expensive and time consuming. Consequently, a variety of quantitative and semiquantitative screening methods have been devised (Table 1.1). Whilst the precision of these semiquantitative methods is less than that of the quantitative methods, the reduction in time and cost justify their widespread use. Unfortunately, the chemical methods have been disappointing because of the high incidence of false negative results.

TABLE 1.1 Methods used to estimate the bacterial count in screening programmes

Reference	*Year*	*Method*
Quantitative methods		
Miles and Misra[48]	1938	Pour plate method
Norden and Kass[2]	1968	Surface colony counting
Semiquantitative methods		
Andriole[54]	1975	Wire loop method
Guttman and Naylor[51]	1967	Dipslide
Bradley *et al.*[55]	1967	Swab method
Leigh and Williams[56]	1964	Filter paper method
Chemical methods		
Smith *et al.*[57]	1961	The Greiss nitrite test
Schersten and Fritz[58]	1967	Reduction of urinary glucose
Simmons and Williams[59]	1962	Tetrazolium chloride reduction

Justification of screening

30% of women with ASB in pregnancy develop acute pyelonephritis. These women are often severely debilitated by their illness and may require hospital admission, intravenous fluids and drugs. Some women develop preterm labour during acute febrile episodes and there is an increased risk of sepsis in the infant. In addition, bacteriuria in pregnancy has been linked with anaemia, low birthweight and toxaemia[60]. Although it is not clear if all these problems can be prevented by treatment of ASB, there is clear evidence that the incidence of acute pyelonephritis can be reduced by treatment[60–63]. Wilson and Jungner[64] suggested that in order for a screening programme to be worthwhile, four criteria must be fulfilled:

(1) The condition sought must be an important health hazard.
(2) A latent phase must be recognizable by a simple test.
(3) The natural history and benefits of treatment must be known.
(4) The cost of identification and treatment of cases must be economically balanced against the expenditure on medical care as a whole.

Screening for bacteriuria during pregnancy would appear to fulfil these criteria. The cost benefit has been evaluated by Asscher[19] who estimated that, in 1975, there would be a net saving to the Health Service of £1 250 000 if all women in England and Wales were screened. Recently, the opposite view has been advocated[65]. The authors argue that 70% of women were receiving antibiotic therapy unnecessarily. Williams[33] also made this point and was able to identify those most at risk of developing acute pyelonephritis by their poor concentrating ability and raised level of antibodies to infecting organisms. These women were also most likely to undergo relapse or reinfection following treatment with a short course of antibiotic. In practice, most obstetricians have opted for screening and treatment of ASB. In the event that the prevalence of ASB were much lower than 5%, the benefits of screening would be less and a greater proportion of cases of acute pyelonephritis would occur amongst those women who had not had bacteriuria at the time of screening. Whilst the benefit to individuals who underwent screening and treatment would remain, the cost benefit would be considerably reduced. In these arguments, the benefit to the infant has rarely been considered. There are now data from more than one study which suggest that bacteriuria may be detrimental to the health of the fetus[61,66] and acute pyelonephritis is associated with an increased risk of prematurity and sepsis in the infant[67,68]. Some of the effects on the fetus or infant are preventable by treatment and this offers the strongest argument in favour of screening.

Prevalence of bacteriuria

There have been many studies of ASB in both pregnant and non-pregnant women (Table 1.2). The prevalence in pregnant women has been shown to be between 3.5% and 8%. This is comparable to the prevalence of ASB in non-pregnant women, but higher than that seen in schoolgirls[74] or nuns[73] suggesting that sexual activity may be a factor[15]. ASB is an intermittent condition and may resolve as a result of spontaneous cure or following the administration of antibiotics which may have been given for an unrelated condition. Reinfection is common in women prone to bacteriuria and some women are exposed to ASB either continuously or intermittently from childhood[75]. It seems likely that the majority of women with ASB in pregnancy had infected urine before the onset of pregnancy. Although it has been stated that ASB does not resolve spontaneously in pregnancy[76], there is little hard evidence to support this view. Because of the relatively

TABLE 1.2 Prevalence of bacteriuria in females

Reference	*Mode of urine collection*	*Year*	*Prevalence*
Pregnancy			
Kass[63]	MSU × 2	1960	6–7%
Kincaid Smith and Bullen[62]	MSU × 2	1965	6%
Williams[33]	MSU × 2	1970	3.8%
Kaitz and Hodder[69]	MSU × 2	1961	4.4%
Turck *et al.*[70]	CSU	1962	6.5%
McFadyen *et al.*[71]	SPA	1973	6.6%
Adult women			
Sussman *et al.*[72]	MSU × 2	1969	3.5%
Kass *et al.*[49]	MSU × 2	1965	5.0%
Nuns			
Kunin and McCormack[73]	MSU × 2	1968	0.5–1%
Schoolgirls			
Kunin *et al.*[74]	MSU × 2	1961	1.2%

MSU = midstream urine
CSU = catheter specimen of urine
SPA = suprapubic aspiration of urine

short duration of pregnancy, only a fraction of those women who might have spontaneous remissions of bacteriuria actually do so during pregnancy. Henderson and Reinke showed that only 57% of untreated negro women who had ASB at the first antenatal visit still had bacteriuria at 38 weeks[47].

Relationship with age, parity, social class and race

Kass[5], Stuart *et al.*[77], Whalley[78] and Savage *et al.*[79] found that the prevalence of ASB increased with age and parity whilst Kaitz and Hodder[69], Turck *et al.*[70] and Layton[80] showed an increased prevalence with parity alone which was more marked among negroes. Turner[81], Sleigh *et al.*[82] and Williams *et al.*[83] were unable to demonstrate any relationship with age or parity. Little[61] found the prevalence of bacteriuria decreased with increasing age but was higher in multiparous women. Patrick[84] and Williams[33] also found bacteriuria significantly more common in the youngest women. Williams *et al.* were able to show a relationship with social class, with women from higher social class being less likely to have ASB than women of low social class[85]. This finding confirmed previous results from Kaitz and Hodder[69], Henderson *et al.*[86], Turck *et al.*[70], Monto and Rantz[87], and Layton[80]. There is a close relationship between age and parity which is influenced by social class and race. This complex relationship and the fact that some surveys were carried out in hospitals where there may have been a bias in patient selection, may account for some of the differences observed. Some authors found a slight excess of black women with ASB but there is a possibility that this is due to an excess in lower social economic and high parity groups.

Bacteriology

Escherichia coli is the commonest bacterial pathogen in pregnancy[33,62,63]. *Klebsiella spp.* are renowned for causing acute pyelonephritis in pregnancy and have been found in 2–30% of cultures. Proteus accounted for 7% in Williams' study[33] (1970), but are less common in other series. Criteria for the significance of colony counts for Gram positive organisms have not been clearly established[88,89], but Meijers-Sever (1979) found anaerobic bacteria in urine obtained by suprapubic aspiration and claimed that these organisms are often present in the urine of healthy pregnant women[90]. McDowall *et al.* found anaerobic and other fastidious organisms in asymptomatic pregnant women[91]. *Staphylococcus saprophylicus* is responsible for some symptomatic urinary tract infections but its role in asymptomatic infection is less clear. Recently *Ureaplasma urealyticum* and *Gardnerella vaginalis* have been found in women with pre-eclampsia[92].

Radiological findings

The prevalence of radiological abnormalities of the upper urinary tract in women with ASB has been reported as being between 17 and 50%. In a prospective study of bacteriuria in pregnant women in Cardiff, Williams *et al.* (1968) found that 17 of 100 (17%) women had evidence of renal scarring, and, in 10 (10%), vesicoureteric reflux was present 4–6 monthly postpartum[93]. Half of the women with vesicoureteric reflux had scarred kidneys. Bladder diverticula were noted in 11 women, 7 of whom had no other significant abnormalities. Ureteric dilatation was noted in 10 women, 2 of whom had bladder diverticula. The prevalence and distribution of these radiological abnormalities were similar to those found in 5–11-year-old bacteriuric schoolgirls identified in the Cardiff/Oxford bacteriuria survey[94]. Two women were found to have renal calculi. Both had scarred kidneys and one had vesicoureteric reflux. Kincaid Smith and Bullen found a slightly higher proportion of radiological abnormalities[62]. In their series of 134 women, 50% had significant abnormalities on the pyelogram, chronic pyelonephritis was present in 9.7%, probable chronic pyelonephritis was present in 8.2%, and a further 8.2% had calyceal abnormalities consistent with papillary necrosis or analgesic nephropathy. Renal calculi were present in 7.5%; 11.9% had miscellaneous abnormalities, including tuberculosis and hydronephrosis. Five of the women in their study underwent surgery for obstruction or poor function of one kidney. In one case, infection was superimposed on a tuberculous kidney, and, in another four, obstruction was due to renal calculi. There is, however, a possibility that, in this hospital-based study, there is bias in the selection of cases referred. The Cardiff study, which included all women in the city undergoing pregnancy during a 12-month period, and included both hospital, nursing home and home deliveries, may be more representative of the population as a whole.

Complications of bacteriuria in pregnancy

Complications of ASB include acute pyelonephritis, anaemia, toxaemia, prematurity and an increased perinatal mortality. The extent to which these events can be related to ASB itself or to underlying renal abnormalities has remained controversial in spite of numerous studies. Differences in populations studied and in the design of studies may be responsible for some of the conflicting results obtained.

Acute pyelonephritis: relationship with bacteriuria and treatment

Acute pyelonephritis (bacteriuria with fever and loin pain) occurs in approximately 1% of pregnancies, but, amongst women with asymptomatic bacteriuria, acute pyelonephritis may occur in 23–43% if left untreated. Kass suggested that, if all pregnant women with asymptomatic bacteriuria were treated, acute pyelonephritis would be almost totally eliminated[63], and, in one study, he treated bacteriuric women with sulphamethoxypyridoxine, 0.5 g daily, from soon after diagnosis to term[95]. No patient treated in this study developed acute pyelonephritis. Other workers have been less successful. In the study of Kincaid Smith and Bullen in 1965, women with ASB were treated with sulphonamides unless the organism was resistant in which case ampicillin was used[62]. Nitrofurantoin was used when there was resistance to ampicillin. They found that 3% of treated bacteriuric women developed acute pyelonephritis compared with 37% in the untreated group. A similar result was achieved by Little (1966) who used antibiotics for several weeks[61]. In this study, acute pyelonephritis developed in 0.4% of women who did not have bacteriuria at the time of screening. Williams *et al.*[83] used short courses of treatment with sulphonamide initially; 78% of women had sterile urine one week after completion of treatment. Women in whom infection was still present had a second course of either sulphonamide, ampicillin or tetracycline for 7 days. Those who failed to respond to two courses of treatment were unlikely to respond to further courses. A high proportion of this group had radiological abnormalities and developed symptomatic infection. In the study by Savage *et al.* (1967), women were treated with sulphonamides or nitrofurantoin[79]. None of the 75 women in whom the urine was successfully rendered sterile developed acute pyelonephritis but there were 18 who continued to have ASB and one of these developed acute pyelonephritis during pregnancy. In addition, 5 women developed acute pyelonephritis postpartum. One woman had been successfully treated and the other four were from the group in whom treatment had failed.

Kaitz and Hodder (1961) found 12 cases of acute pyelonephritis in a group of 616 women (2%); three cases occurred amongst 17 women with untreated ASB (18%) whereas 9 cases occurred amongst 573 women (1.6%) who did not have evidence of ASB at initial screening[69]. Because some cases of acute pyelonephritis develop in women who do not have bacteriuria at the start of pregnancy, it is unlikely that acute pyelonephritis will be completely eliminated by screening and treatment. Women with ASB and sickle cell trait have an increased risk of developing acute pyelonephritis[96].

Anaemia

The relationship between ASB, underlying functional abnormalities and anaemia is controversial, several studies having yielded conflicting results. Giles and Brown[97], Layton[80] and Patrick[84] all noted an increased incidence of anaemia in bacteriuric women when compared with non-bacteriuric women, but Kaitz and Hodder[69], Little[61], Savage *et al.*[79] and Condie *et al.*[98] were unable to show a significant difference in haemoglobin level. In a large prospective study in which women in London and Birmingham were screened for ASB and randomly allocated to treatment or placebo, there was a small difference in mean haemoglobin level at initial assessment, the mean for women with bacteriuria being 78.5% compared with 80.2% for controls[76]. At 32 weeks of gestation the difference was smaller, 77.1% for bacteriuric women compared with 78.8% for controls. However, at this point in pregnancy, significantly more women in the placebo-treated bacteriuric group were anaemic (Hb 70%) 21.8% *vs.* 14.6% of the groups studied. This increase in anaemic women is largely accounted for by an excess of women in the bacteriuric group with haemoglobin levels of 60–70% and may represent a subgroup who developed complications during pregnancy or who had underlying renal disease. Amongst women with ASB, there was no significant difference in mean haemoglobin levels between treated and untreated women although more untreated women became anaemic during pregnancy. The incidence of anaemia is reduced by treatment. They showed that the highest incidence of anaemia (45%) was in untreated bacteriuric women who developed acute pyelonephritis and were given antibiotics at that stage.

Toxaemia

The relationship between bacteriuria and the subsequent development of hypertension and proteinuria (or toxaemia of pregnancy) remains controversial. Stuart *et al.*[99], Kincaid Smith and Bullen[62] and Norden and Kilpatrick[100] all found an increase in the incidence of pre-eclamptic toxaemia whilst Bryant *et al.*[101], Low *et al.*[102], Little[61], Condie *et al.*[98], Williams *et al.*[103] and Williams[76] were unable to show any association with hypertension or toxaemia. These conflicting results may be related to the way in which women are referred for hospital delivery, some centres attracting women who are expected to have complicated pregnancies. Although Kincaid Smith and Bullen[62] were able to show that women with ASB in their series were at greater risk of developing pre-eclampsia, their group of women also had the highest rate of renal parenchymal abnormalities. They were unable to show that treatment reduced the rate of pre-eclampsia and this would be consistent with the hypothesis that hypertension and proteinuria developed as a complication of the underlying renal disease rather than as a result of bacteriuria. Further evidence to support this association is obtained from the observations of Becker *et al.*[9] that women with reflux nephropathy were inclined to develop severe hypertension and proteinuria during pregnancy. Ihle, Long and Oats observed that women with significant underlying renal disease were inclined to develop pre-eclampsia before 37 weeks gestation[104]. Fifty-two pregnancies have been studied in 34 women from the Cardiff/Oxford bacteriuria survey[105]. These women had bacteriuria in childhood and were followed prospectively. Although 35% of women had evidence of ASB at the start of pregnancy, all those women who remained bacteriuric were given appropriate treatment. Hypertension and proteinuria developed in 1 of 36 pregnancies in women with radiologically normal kidneys and in 5 of 16 pregnancies in women with scarred kidneys ($p<0.01$). This data also suggests that it is the underlying renal disease rather than ASB which predisposes to this complication.

Effect on renal function

Apart from altered micturition patterns, there is no reason to think that ASB confined to the bladder affects renal function. Unfortunately, it is not possible to distinguish on clinical grounds between upper and lower urinary tract infection in asymptomatic women. There is good evidence that upper tract infection interferes significantly with renal function both in symptomatic and asymptomatic individuals. In 1961, Kaitz observed a reduction in renal concentrating capacity in half of the women with asymptomatic bacteriuria in his study[7]. This was confirmed in 1965 by Norden and Tuttle who were able to reverse this abnormality with antibiotic treatment and eradication of bacteriuria[106]. Elder and Kass[107] found similar results but also noted that it was most often untreated bacteriuric women with poor concentrating capacity who went on to develop acute pyelonephritis. Williams[108] showed that the maximum urine osmolality in pregnant bacteriuric women became lower as pregnancy progressed, whilst, in non-bacteriuric women, the maximum urine osmolality increased. There was a significant positive correlation between the maximum urine osmolality and creatinine clearance. Creatinine clearance in bacteriuric women fell slightly as pregnancy progressed and was significantly lower when carried out under conditions of fluid restriction. This fall is not seen in non-bacteriuric women. Harris[109] also found that women with renal ASB, as judged by a positive fluorescent antibody test, had lower creatinine clearances than women in whom only lower tract infection was present. Whalley, Cunningham and Martin showed that there was a transient fall in glomerular filtration rate during attacks of acute pyelonephritis in pregnancy[8].

Davison, Sprott and Selkon[110] found that women who had had untreated childhood bacteriuria but radiologically normal kidneys had lower values of tubular glucose reabsorption than women in whom bacteriuria had been treated in childhood or healthy controls. None of these women were bacteriuric at the time of the study. He also found that these women had a smaller increase in glomerular filtration rate during pregnancy than expected. Similar abnormalities were found in women with renal scarring who had received two years prophylactic antimicrobial therapy during childhood. Their study suggested that ASB in childhood caused proximal tubular damage which was unmasked by the physiological demands of pregnancy.

Effect on the infant

There is clear evidence that ASB has an adverse effect on the fetus. Kass *et al.* reported a perinatal mortality rate of 17% amongst bacteriuric women and showed that this could be reduced to 10% by treatment[49]. He also found an increased incidence of small infants, a tendency which could be reversed by treatment. Although in other studies results have been less clear cut there is a large body of data to suggest that maternal ASB has an adverse effect on the infant. The effects on the infant are discussed in greater depth at the end of the chapter.

Effect of treatment on asymptomatic bacteriuria

In early studies, a wide variety of drugs were used to treat ASB with a varying degree of success. Drugs included sulphonamides, ampicillin, nitrofurantoin, cycloserine and even tetracycline, a drug which would not now be considered for use during pregnancy because of its accumulation in bones and teeth[33,62,83,95]. In some instances, short courses of antimicrobial drugs were used whilst in others long-term treatment was used until after delivery, either in full dosage or as low-dose prophylaxis. In all studies where appropriate samples were taken, the urine was rendered sterile soon after initiation of therapy but reinfection was common, occurring in a third of cases where short courses of treatment were used. Those women who became reinfected most often were most likely to develop acute pyelonephritis and other complications of bacteriuria and were also most likely to have radiological abnormalities and abnormalities of renal function. The effect of treatment of ASB on the complication rate has been discussed in the appropriate sections.

CLINICAL ASPECTS

Although much information has been acquired from prospective studies based on screening programmes, in routine clinical practice, management is tailored to the needs of the individual patient. The case for routine screening for ASB has been made and many obstetric units regard this as normal clinical practice. Symptomatic urinary tract infection is common, but must be differentiated from other conditions which can give rise to dysuria and frequency. Acute pyelonephritis is essentially a clinical diagnosis in a febrile patient supported by appropriate urinary findings. Prompt treatment with an antibiotic regarded as safe in pregnancy combined with supportive treatment is essential.

Urine culture and microscopy

Although women with ASB usually have a bacterial colony count of >100 000 cfu/ml, and, for epidemiological purposes, this figure identifies those women who probably have ASB, the situation in clinical practice is slightly different. There are fewer data for the reliability of the colony count from mid-stream samples during acute symptomatic infection[111] and Stamm *et al.*[112] have pointed out the pitfalls of relying too heavily on the colony count. In addition, there are a number of factors which may lower the colony count. Frequent bladder emptying will eliminate more organisms and the production of large volumes of urine will dilute the viable count. Very dilute urine, such as may be produced as a result of acute pyelonephritis, creates conditions which are less favourable for bacterial growth. It has been clearly established in infants that counts as low as 1000 may occur with acute pyelonephritis[113].

In the presence of acute pyelonephritis, the number of pus cells in the urine is increased. Pus cells correlate poorly with ASB and have tended to be ignored in epidemiological studies. Their presence in the clinical setting supports the diagnosis of urinary tract infection.

Antimicrobials given prior to collection of the sample will kill organisms, lowering the count or rendering urine sterile. Organisms may be seen on microscopy although there is no growth.

Tests of localization

When a pregnant woman presents with fever, loin pain, bacteriuria and pyuria, there is little doubt that she has upper tract infection. In the presence of less dramatic symptoms or ASB, it is difficult or impossible to differentiate on purely clinical grounds whether or not the upper tract is involved. Infection involving the upper tract is more likely to recur and may be an indication of underlying renal disease. Thus, knowledge of upper tract involvement influences management and prognosis. Tests of localization have never been entirely reliable and are used more in research programmes than in clinical practice.

Ureteric catheterization has generally been regarded as the standard test for localization against which other methods have been tested. Whilst this technique is straight forward in theory, in practice, it is invasive and not entirely without risk. It has the advantage that the side of the infection can be localized. False positive results have been obtained when organisms have been carried into the ureter on the catheter or in the presence of vesicoureteric reflux. Fairley *et al.* have described a modification of this technique using only a urethral catheter[114]. After draining the bladder, it is washed out with an antimicrobial agent. Subsequent samples are collected and presumed to represent urine from the upper tracts.

Winberg[115] demonstrated a reversible concentrating defect in children with acute urinary tract infection and proposed that this was evidence of upper tract involvement. Similar observations have been made in pregnant women with ASB[7,106]. Those women with poor concentrating capacity were more likely to develop acute pyelonephritis. During acute pyelonephritis, defective urine-concentrating capacity is always found and improves over a period of days or weeks following treatment. Acute kidney damage causes an increase in enzymes released into the urine. β-Glucuronidase and lactic acid dehydrogenase isoenzyme 5 tend to be raised in the presence of acute pyelonephritis[116]. β-2-microglobulin is a low-molecular-weight protein which is normally absorbed by the renal tubules. During upper tract infection, increased amounts reach the urine. Serum antibodies against the O antigen are raised following acute pyelonephritis and a raised antibody titre correlates to some extent with other tests of upper tract infection[33]. Similarly, antibody can be found coating the bacteria in the urine during upper tract infection[36,109]. Although in clinically obvious cases of acute pyelonephritis there is a good correlation with tests of localization, these tests have a poorer predictive value in level diagnosis in ASB.

Clinical presentations

Symptoms of lower urinary tract infection are common in pregnancy although bacterial urinary tract infection may account for only a small proportion of women with these symptoms. Frequent bladder emptying occurs from early on in pregnancy and may be related to the enlarging uterus. Dysuria may be related to local urethral problems and, in the absence of bacterial infection, is known as the 'urethral syndrome'. *Chlamydia trachomatis* has been implicated in this condition[117]. Vaginal discharge or perineal soreness can also mimic the symptoms of cystitis or lower urinary tract infection. Bladder infection may resolve spontaneously, become asymptomatic or resolve following antimicrobial treatment.

Acute pyelonephritis has already been mentioned several times in this chapter. It may arise with sterile urine at the start of pregnancy but most cases arise in women with ASB. It is rare for a pregnant woman with acute lower tract symptoms to progress to acute pyelonephritis. Women with ASB have few symptoms of lower tract infection but present suddenly in the second or third trimester with florid symptoms. Fever, malaise and systemic symptoms may precede the loin pain so that urinary infection is not immediately suspected. Eventually, pain is localized to one or other flank and loin tenderness can be elicited. It is usually difficult to feel the kidneys because of the large uterus. Occasionally bacteraemia or septicaemia may occur. The latter is more likely in the presence of an obstructive lesion or renal stones. The development of septicaemia, recurrent, severe (relapsing) infection or failure to respond within 48 h to the appropriate antibiotic would be an indication for further investigation to exclude obstruction. In the presence of serious illness, the risk to the infant of a limited intravenous pyelogram is less than the risk of failing to diagnose and treat an obstructive lesion giving rise to recurrent upper tract infection with all its attendant risks. With the widespread availability of ultrasound, obstruction can be ruled out without resort to X rays although it can be difficult to differentiate between obstruction and physiological dilatation, and a plain X ray is required to show radio-opaque calculi.

Recurrent infection

Recurrence of urinary tract infection may be due to reinfection or to a relapse of a partially treated infection[118]. In most cases, the urine is rendered sterile during and after treatment with an antibiotic to which the organism is sensitive. Reinfection with a new organism is a common event in women prone to ASB or recurrent symptomatic infection. It is not possible to differentiate between reinfections with a similar organism and a relapse of a partially treated infection. The latter is more likely to occur following upper tract infection particularly if there is an underlying renal abnormality and if the antibiotic treatment was given for only a few days. Rarely, the urine remains infected throughout treatment (persisting infection), in which case a significant renal lesion should be suspected.

Obstruction, stones, perinephric abscess

Obstruction may develop due to stones or may come to light because infection develops in an already abnormal urinary tract. Congenital lesions, such as pelviureteric junction obstruction or less commonly vesicoureteric junction obstruction, may present with acute pyelonephritis in pregnancy. Women who have undergone reimplantation of the ureter for vesicoureteric reflux have been known to develop transient ureteric obstruction when the ureter becomes stretched over the broad ligament. Once obstruction has been diagnosed, some form of drainage procedure will be required. The use of a percutaneous nephrostomy or pigtail catheters until after delivery of the infant usually avoids the need for surgery until full investigation and treatment can be carried out. Infection when associated with renal calculi can be difficult or impossible to eradicate. Such women will almost certainly have recurrent episodes of upper tract infection. Symptoms can often be kept at bay by prolonged courses of antibiotic therapy, but this in itself is undesirable because of the effect any drug might have on the fetus. In this difficult situation, the clinician will almost certainly find it necessary to use repeated courses of treatment for repeated attacks of pyelonephritis. If obstruction occurs, free drainage must be established. Occasionally, surgical stone removal may have to be considered during pregnancy.

The finding of sterile urine and a normal urinary deposit in the face of symptoms and signs of acute pyelonephritis is a rare occurrence which should lead the clinician to suspect total ureteric obstruction on one side or a perinephric abscess. Ultrasound will help to establish the diagnosis and drainage of pus is mandatory if further problems are to be avoided. Egwnata described an unusual case in which a pyelonephrosis ruptured into the peritoneum[119].

Management of infection

When prescribing during pregnancy, consideration must be given to the altered physiological state and increased glomerular filtration rate, as well as the effect of the drug on the fetus. The principles have been discussed by Rubin[120] and Wise[121]. At the time of conception and during the first trimester, it is particularly important to avoid any drug which might have a teratogenic effect. Later in pregnancy, drugs which might have an adverse effect on the fetus after delivery should be avoided. Most drugs cross the placenta and are excreted in breastmilk. When treating clinical infection, it is often necessary to initiate antibiotic therapy before the results of culture are available. As most infections are due to Gram negative organisms, a broad spectrum antibiotic should be used. If the woman is significantly ill with acute pyelonephritis, intravenous antibiotics will be required. If necessary, the antibiotic can be changed when the sensitivity of the organism is known. Provided the organism is sensitive to the antibiotic, clinical improvement should occur within 48 h. Failure to improve by 72 h should lead one to suspect that the organism is not sensitive to the antibiotic chosen or an underlying obstructive lesion which requires urgent drainage. It is important to ensure an adequate fluid intake since there will be excessive losses due to sweating and loss of renal concentrating capacity. Dehydration may be exacerbated by vomiting and anorexia. Paracetamol may be used as an antipyretic and analgesic.

Although prophylactic treatment with low-dose trimethoprim or nitrofurantoin are effective in preventing recurrent bacteriuria in non-pregnant women, experience is limited in pregnancy. It is undesirable to expose the fetus to a prolonged course of antibiotic and it may be wiser to rely on regular urine culture with short courses of treatment when necessary. Following acute pyelonephritis, there is a high risk of further attacks[122]. Williams has advocated continuous prophylaxis for women with recurrent bacteriuria after several courses of therapy[83]. Single-dose treatment has been advocated by Bailey who found that women with normal urinary tracts developed sterile urine, whereas women with underlying abnormalities relapsed or became re-infected[123]. Thus, single-dose treatment had the advantages of lower side effects in the mother, less drug exposure to the fetus and a means by which those women who had underlying disease could be identified.

Choice of antibiotic

Sulphonamides have been used in pregnancy for many years. They may be expected to eradicate 50–70% of urinary tract infections. There does not appear to be any untoward effect on the fetus *in utero* although sulphonamides readily cross the placenta. After delivery, sulphonamides acquired from the maternal circulation can increase the risk of kernicterus by displacing bilirubin from its binding sites. In addition, problems have been encountered from the Stevens–Johnson syndrome and neonatal jaundice due to glucose-6-phosphate dehydrogenese deficiency.

Ampicillin has not been shown to be associated with any adverse effects on the fetus and consequently this is the drug of choice for urinary infection in pregnancy. It can be given intravenously but has the drawback that only 60% of organisms will be sensitive so that it is not the drug of choice for seriously ill patients in whom sensitivity is not known. Other drawbacks include maternal diarrhoea and vaginal thrush.

Cephalosporins are related to the penicillins and are also acceptable in pregnancy, although they produce similar side effects. A higher proportion of Gram-negative organisms will be sensitive to the cephalosporins than ampicillin.

Trimethoprim and cotrimoxazole are effective in the management of urinary tract infection and the side effects are fewer than with ampicillin or cephalexin. These drugs have not been used extensively in pregnancy and there are insufficient data to recommend their use with confidence. The antifolate effect of trimethoprim may be detrimental to both the mother and the fetus. The sulphonamide component of cotrimoxazole, sulphamethoxazole, will give rise to all the problems already described for sulphonamides.

Aminoglycosides are important and potent parenteral drugs that are useful in the management of the sick patient. Their broad spectrum and bactericidal effects give them advantages over other drugs, even though they are not without risk and must be given intravenously. There is no doubt that they cross the placenta easily and toxicity to the eighth nerve of the fetus has been reported after streptomycin[124]. Gentamicin and netilmicin are widely used for their broad spectrum against a variety of organisms and tobramycin is effective against

Pseudomonas spp. Drug levels should be monitored and the dose should be modified in the presence of renal failure. Because of their broad spectrum, these drugs may be used initially in severe cases of acute pyelonephritis, changing to a less toxic drug if possible when bacterial sensitivity is known.

Nitrofurantoin has had widespread use in the management of ASB or lower tract symptomatic infection. It is effective and apparently free from teratogenic effects. It does, however, give rise to a number of adverse effects in the mother, including nausea, vomiting, pulmonary fibrosis, liver damage, blood dyscrasias and, in those with impaired renal function, neuropathy. The more serious side effects are related to prolonged usage and are uncommon. In addition, it does not give rise to high tissue levels and is not thought to be satisfactory for the treatment of acute pyelonephritis.

Tetracycline causes abnormalities of teeth and bone development as well as hepatotoxicity in the mother and should be avoided.

Chloramphenicol is rarely required for the management of urinary infection and may give rise to blood dyscrasias in the mother and grey syndrome in the infant.

The new quinolone derivatives are effective in urinary infection outside pregnancy but are not thought to be safe in pregnancy. They accumulate in cartilage and may cause damage to the fetus.

Postpartum infection

In Williams' study[33], 97 of 207 (47%) women with ASB at the antenatal clinic had ASB on the 7th day postpartum. The practice of catheterization in relation to obstetric manoeuvers (forceps delivery and caesarian section) and postpartum to relieve urinary retention also contributes to postpartum infection. Turck and Petersdorf showed that the incidence of infection following catheterization could be reduced significantly by a short course of sulphonamide[10]. Similar results were shown with nitrofurantoin, ampicillin and cotrimoxazole[16]. Acute pyelonephritis is common in the puerperium but the risk decreases with time from delivery.

THE INFANT

There is an increasing volume of evidence to suggest that urinary infection in its various clinical presentations may be detrimental to the infant. The stormy course of the woman described in the introduction illustrates some of the problems encountered 50 years ago[4]. It was difficult to ascertain whether problems were due to the prolonged illness of acute pyelonephritis, high fever, hypertension or underlying renal disease. Nevertheless, descriptions of spontaneous abortion, preterm labour and small infants are common. Kass reported a remarkably high perinatal mortality of 17% in untreated bacteriuric women and found a dramatic improvement in treated women[63]. Other workers have also found an excess of perinatal deaths. Leigh and Williams found 4% in a group of 100 bacteriuric women[56] and Layton[80] found 2.9%. Savage *et al.* found 7 perinatal deaths among 72 women who were treated with placebo and no perinatal deaths among treated cases[79]. Similar results were found by Condie *et al.*[98], Gruneberg *et al.*[125] and Little[61]. Kincaid Smith and Bullen showed an increased fetal loss in bacteriuric women but were unable to influence this with antimicrobial therapy[62].

Kass found that 24% of infants born to bacteriuric mothers weighed less than 2500 g. The rate in treated bacteriuric women fell to 10%, a figure similar to that found in non-bacteriuric women. Similar results were found by Le Blanc and McGanity[66], Kincaid Smith and Bullen[62], Stuart *et al.*[77], Layton[80] and Condie *et al.*[98]. Gruneberg *et al.*[125] were unable to show a significant difference between treated bacteriuric women and controls, but further analysis of the treated group showed that the mean birthweight was lowest amongst those women who had persisting infection in spite of several courses of treatment. Several other workers were unable to show a significant difference in birthweight or in the incidence of small infants[47,69,81,100,102].

Sever, Ellenberg and Edmonds[68], using data from the Infectious Diseases Branch and Office of Biometry and Epidemiology, National Institute and Communicative Disorders and Stroke, found that there was an increased risk of low birthweight infants and still birth amongst women with urinary infection in pregnancy. They also noted an increased risk of rhesus incompatibility and eye infection, although it is difficult to see how these conditions could be influenced by maternal urinary tract infection. In addition they found that the motor development of these infants at 8 months was significantly behind that of controls. Naeye[67] and Naeye *et al.*[126] also studied data from the same source. They found that the perinatal mortality rate for common conditions (amniotic fluid infection, congenital malformations, placental infarction, abruptio placentae, growth retarded placentae, and placenta praevia) was significantly greater if the mother had laboratory evidence to suggest urinary tract infection, although the prevalence of all but one of these conditions was not significantly different in bacteriuric women and controls. This data is interesting because it suggests that much of the reported increase in perinatal loss may occur because maternal urinary tract infection makes the fetus less able to cope with adverse events in pregnancy. The only condition which occurred with increased frequency was placental growth retardation. McGrady *et al.* found that the fetal mortality rate was 2.4 times the rate for the whole population and low birthweight infants occurred significantly more often in pregnancies associated with acute urinary tract infection[127].

A recent study of pregnant women known to have had asymptomatic bacteriuria in childhood showed that their infants had significantly lower Apgar scores than controls[105]. Only 35% of these women were bacteriuric at the start of pregnancy and all those in whom bacteriuria was confirmed received appropriate treatment. Patrick[128] studied 133 bacteriuric women, 58 of whom were successfully treated. She found no difference in the incidence of spontaneous abortion or stillbirth when compared with 500 controls but neonatal deaths were more common amongst bacteriuric women. The increased mortality was largely accounted for by a higher incidence of midline defect (3.8% *vs.* 0.2%). She found that the infants were more prone to bacteriuria even if the mother had been successfully treated. Four of 8 women who were bacteriuric at term had *Escherichia coli* in the amniotic fluid. Six of 19 blood cultures from umbilical arteries were positive compared with 0 of 20 controls. Ives, Abbott and Bailey[129] also found an increased incidence of amniotic fluid infection in infants born to women with urinary infection.

ADVICE, FAMILY PLANNING AND GENETIC COUNSELLING

With well-developed health care services, there are ample opportunities for counselling women with recurrent urinary infection, vesicoureteric reflux and reflux nephropathy about the implications of their condition and its treatment in relation to family planning.

Oral contraceptives are widely used and the newer, lower dose preparations are relatively free from side effects. Antibiotics can interfere with the absorption of oral contraceptives and women prone to recurrent infection should be warned of this risk[130]. Women with reflux nephropathy are at increased risk of hypertension[131] and this risk will be further increased by oral contraceptives[132]. However, there is no reason why these drugs should not be used provided the risks are explained and regular blood pressure monitoring carried out. If hypertension develops, oral contraceptives should be stopped or a change made to a lower dose or progesterone-only preparation. Rarely, antihypertensive drugs may be used if oral contraceptives are the only acceptable method in a hypertensive woman.

Some sexually active women develop recurrent episodes of symptomatic infection and are managed either with frequent intermittent short courses of antibiotic or long-term low-dose prophylaxis. Trimethoprim and cotrimoxazole are effective drugs for this purpose. However, it is theoretically undesirable to plan a pregnancy whilst taking any drug, particularly folate antagonists. Under these circumstances, the woman should be advised to stop treatment prior to conception. Short courses of ampicillin could be used if really necessary or, alternatively, symptomatic relief could be obtained with potassium citrate mixture.

All women with a past history of reflux, reflux nephropathy, ASB or symptomatic urinary tract infection are at increased risk of ASB and acute pyelonephritis during pregnancy. Such women are only too willing to attend clinic regularly and provide a mid-stream sample if the need for this has been explained. Women with reflux nephropathy are at increased risk of hypertension and proteinuria[105] and, if renal function is impaired, there is a risk that pregnancy might hasten the decline of renal function[9]. Here the importance of planning pregnancies is clear since each pregnancy carries some maternal risk and will probably involve prolonged hospital admission. These women should be advised of the risks of pregnancy and may wish to limit their families to one or two children.

It is now clear that vesicoureteric reflux is familial[133] and the risk to an infant if one parent has reflux or reflux nephropathy is 50%. In addition, there is an increased risk that infants born to women with ASB will have urinary infection themselves[134]. Vesicoureteric reflux can be detected by micturating cystography and infection prevented by prophylactic antimicrobial agents[135]. The symptoms of urinary infection in infants are non-specific and illness may be mild or severe. These women should be warned of the increased risk of urinary tract infection so that the infant's urine can be examined in the event of jaundice, fever, vomiting, weight loss or any unexplained illness, and early treatment initiated in the event of urinary tract infection so that renal scarring can be prevented.

REFERENCES

1. Asscher, A.W., Verrier Jones, K. and Harber, M.J. (1985). An assessment of the need for screening and treatment of covert urinary tract infections. In Asscher, A.W. and Brumfitt, W. (eds.) *Microbial Diseases in Nephrology*, pp. 83–103. (Chichester: John Wiley and Sons)
2. Norden, C.W. and Kass, E.H. (1968). Bacteriuria in pregnancy: A critical appraisal. *Annu. Rev. Med.*, **19**, 413–470
3. Kass, E.H. and Zinner Z.H. (1973). Bacteriuria and pyelonephritis in pregnancy. In Charles, D. and Finland, M. (eds.) *Obstetric and Perinatal Infections*, pp. 407–446; (Philadelphia: Lea Febiger)
4. Weiss, S. and Parker, F. (1939). Pyelonephritis: Its relation to vascular lesions and to arterial hypertension. *Medicine* (*Baltimore*), **18**, 221–315
5. Kass, E.H. (1956). Asymptomatic infections of the urinary tract. *Trans. Assoc. Am. Physicians*, **69**, 56–64
6. Olling, S., Verrier Jones, K., Mackenzie, R., Verrier Jones, E.R., Hanson, L.A. and Asscher, A.W. (1981). A four-year follow-up of schoolgirls with untreated covert bacteriuria: bacteriological aspects. *Clin. Nephrol.*, **16**, 169–171
7. Kaitz, A.L. (1961). Urinary concentrating ability in pregnant women with asymptomatic bacteriuria. *J. Clin. Invest.*, **40**, 1331–1333
8. Whalley, P.J., Cunningham, F.G. and Martin, F.G. (1975). Transient renal dysfunction associated with acute pyelonephritis of pregnancy. *Obstet. Gynecol.*, **46**, 174–177
9. Becker, G.J., Ihle, B.U., Fairley, K.F., Bastos, M. and Kincaid Smith, P. (1986). Effect of pregnancy on moderate renal failure in reflux nephropathy. *Br. Med. J.*, **292**, 796–798

10. Turck, M. and Petersdorf, R.G. (1962). A study of chemoprophylaxis of post-partum urinary tract infection. *J. Am. Med. Assoc.*, **182,** 899–903
11. Gruneberg, R.N., Leigh, D.A. and Brumfitt, W. (1968). *Escherichia coli* serotypes in urinary tract infection: Studies in domiciliary, antenatal and hospital practice. In O'Grady, F. and Brumfitt, W. (eds.) *Urinary Tract Infection*, pp. 68–79. (London: Oxford University Press)
12. Winberg, J. (1986). Balance between host defence and bacterial virulence in urinary tract infection. In Asscher, A.W. and Brumfitt, W. (eds.) *Microbial Diseases in Nephrology*, pp. 197–223. (Chichester: John Wiley and Sons Ltd.)
13. Stamey, T.A. and Sexton, C.C. (1975). The role of vaginal colonisation with enterobacteria in recurrent urinary infections. *J. Urol.*, **113,** 214–217
14. Stamey, T.A., Wehner, N. and Mihara, G. (1978). The immunological basis of recurrent bacteriuria: role of cervico-vaginal antibody in enterobacterial colonization of the introital mucosa. *Medicine (Baltimore)*, **57,** 47–56
15. Buckley, R.M. Jr., McGuckin, M. and MacGregor, R.R. (1978). Urine bacterial counts after sexual intercourse. *N. Engl. J. Med.*, **298,** 321–324
16. Harris, R.E. (1979). Post partum urinary retention: Role of antimicrobial therapy. *Am. J. Obstet. Gynecol.*, **133,** 174–175
17. Roberts, A.P. and Beard, R.W. (1965). Some factors affecting bacterial invasion of the bladder during pregnancy. *Lancet*, **1,** 1133–1136
18. Harber, M.J. and Asscher, A.W. (1985). The virulence of urinary pathogens. *Kidney Int.*, **28,** 717–721
19. Asscher, A.W. (1980). *The Challenge of Urinary Tract Infection*. (London: Academic Press)
20. Asscher, A.W. (1966). Urine as a medium for bacterial growth. *Lancet*, **2,** 1037–1041
21. Waters, W.E., Sussman, M. and Asscher, A.W. (1967). A community study of urinary pH and osmolality. *Br. J. Prev. Soc. Med.*, **21,** 129–132
22. Reidasch, G., Heck, P., Rauterberg, E. and Ritz, E. (1983). Does low urinary sIgA predispose to urinary tract infection? *Kidney Int.*, **23,** 754–763
23. Mackintosh, I.P., Watson, B.W. and O'Grady, F. (1975). Theory of hydrokinetic clearance of bacteria from the urinary bladder. *Invest. Urol.*, **12,** 473–478
24. O'Grady, F., Mackintosh, I.P., Greenwood, D. and Watson, B.W. (1973). Treatment of 'bacterial cystitis' in fully automatic mechanical models simulating conditions of bacterial growth in the urinary bladder. *Br. J. Exp. Pathol.*, **54,** 283–290
25. Lee, H.P. and Mengert, W.F. (1934). The effect of pregnancy on the urinary tract. *J. Am. Med. Assoc.*, **102,** 102–107
26. Fainstat, T. (1963). Physiological hydroureter of pregnancy in a 4-legged animal. *Am. J. Obstet. Gynecol.*, **87,** 486–492
27. Harber, M.J., Topley, N., Jenner, D.E., Mackenzie, R.K., Steadman, R., Knowlden, J.M. and Asscher, A.W. (1986). Virulence factors of urinary pathogens in relation to kidney scarring. In Asscher, A.W. and Brumfitt, W. (eds.) *Microbial Diseases in Nephrology*, pp. 69–82. (Chichester: John Wiley and Sons Ltd.)
28. Topley, N., Steadman, R., Mackenzie, R., Davies, M., Williams, J. and Asscher, A.W. (1987). *E. coli* and renal scarring: The role of hydropholicity in the activities of the inflammatory response. *Rev. Infect. Dis.* (In press)
29. Leffler, H. and Svanborg Eden, C. (1980). Chemical identification of a gly-

cosphingolipid receptor for *Escherichia coli* attaching to human urinary tract epithelial cells and agglutinating human erythrocytes. *FESM Microbiol. Lett.*, **8,** 127–134
30. Svanborg Eden, C., Larsson, P. and Lomberg, H. (1980). Attachment of *Proteus miribalis* bacteria to human urinary tract epithelial cells is different from that of *Escherichia coli. Infect. Immun.*, **27,** 804–807
31. Holmgren, J. and Smith, J.W. (1975). Immunological aspects of urinary tract infections. *Prog. Allergy,* **18,** 289–352
32. Vosti, K.L., Monto, A.S. and Rantz, L.A. (1965). Host parasite interaction in patients with infections due to *Escherichia coli,* II. Serological response of the host. *J. Lab. Clin. Med.*, **66,** 613–626
33. Williams, G.L. (1970). Asymptomatic bacteriuria in pregnancy. *MD Thesis*, University of Wales
34. Glynn, A.A., Brumfitt, W. and Howard, C.J. (1971). K-antigens of *Escherichia coli* and renal involvement in urinary tract infections. *Lancet,* **1,** 514–516
35. Burdon, D.W. (1975). Immunological reactions to urinary infection: The nature and function of secretory immunoglobulins. In Innes Williams, D. and Chisholm, G.D. (eds.) *Scientific Foundations of Urology*, pp. 192–196. (London: Heinemann)
36. Thomas, V., Shelokov, A. and Forland, M. (1974). Antibody coated bacteria in the urine and the site of urinary tract infection. *N. Engl. J. Med.*, **290,** 588–590
37. Mattingly, R.F. (1967). The physiology of the urinary tract in pregnancy. In Marcus, S.L. and Marcus, C.C. (eds.) *Advances in Obstetrics and Gynaecology*, pp. 124–136. (Baltimore: Williams and Wilkins)
38. Marchant, D.J. (1972). Effects of pregnancy and progestational agents on the urinary tract. *Am. J. Obstet. Gynecol.*, **112,** 487–501
39. Fainstat, T. (1963). Ureteral dilatation in pregnancy: A review. *Obstet. Gynecol. Surv.*, **18,** 845–860
40. Fairley, K.F., Bond, A.G. and Adey, F.D. (1966). The site of infection in pregnancy bacteriuria. *Lancet,* **1,** 939–41
41. El-Katib, M.T., Becker, G.J. and Kincaid Smith, P.S. (1987). Complications associated with pregnancy in patients with reflux nephropathy. In *Abstract Xth International Society of Nephrology*, pp. 113. (Oxford: Alden Press)
42. Beeson, P.B. and Rowley, D. (1969). The anticomplimentary effect of kidney tissue and its association with ammonia production. *J. Exp. Med.*, **110,** 685–697
43. Chernew, I. and Braude, A.I. (1962). Depression of phagocytosis by solutes in concentrations found in the kidney and urine. *J. Clin. Ivest.*, **41,** 1945–1953
44. Acquatella, H., Little, P.J., de Wardner, H.E. and Coleman, J.C. (1967). The effect of urine osmolality and pH on the bactericidal activity of plasma. *Clin. Sci.*, **33,** 471–480
45. Verrier Jones, K., Asscher, A.W. and Verrier Jones, E.R. (1986). Covert infection in childhood. In Asscher, A.W. and Brumfitt, W. (eds.) *Microbial Diseases in Nephrology*, pp. 225–241. (Chichester: John Wiley and Sons Ltd.)
46. Leading article (1978). Covert bacteriuria – peril or partnership. *Br. Med. J.*, **1,** 1649–1650
47. Henderson, M. and Reinke, W.A. (1965). The relationship betwen bacteriuria and prematurity. In Kass, E.H. (ed.) *Progress in Pyelonephritis*, pp. 27–32. (Philadelphia: F.A. Davis and Co.)

48. Miles, A.A. and Misra, S. (1938). The estimation of bactericidal power of the blood. *J. Hyg.*, **38,** 732–749
49. Kass, E.H., Savage, W. and Santamarina, B.A.G. (1965). The significance of bacteriuria in preventative medicine. In Kass, E.H. (ed.) *Progress in Pyelonephritis*, pp. 3–10. (Philadelphia: F.A. Davis and Co.)
50. Porter, I.A. and Brodie, J. (1969). Boric acid preservation of urine samples. *Br. Med. J.*, **1,** 353–355
51. Guttmann, D.E. and Naylor, G.R.E. (1967). Quantitive urine culture in general practice. *Br. Med. J.*, **3,** 343–345
52. Cowan, S.T. and Steel, K.J. (1965). *Manual for the Identification of Medical Bacteria.* (London: Cambridge University Press)
53. McFadyen, I.R. and Eykyn, S.J. (1968). Suprapubic aspiration of urine in pregnancy. *Lancet*, **1,** 1112–1114
54. Andriole, V.T. (1975). Urinary tract infections in pregnancy. *Urol. Clin. N. Am.*, **2,** 485–498
55. Bradley, J.M., Crowley, N. and Darrell, J.H. (1967). Method for detection of bacteriuria suitable for use in general practice. *Br. Med. J.*, **4,** 649–651
56. Leigh, D.A. and Williams, J.D. (1964). Method for detection of bacteriuria in large groups of patients. *J. Clin. Pathol.*, **17,** 498–503
57. Smith, L.G., Thayer, W.L., Malta, E.M. and Utz, J.P. (1961). Relationship of the Greiss nitrite test to bacterial culture in the diagnosis of urinary infection. *Ann. Intern. Med.*, **54,** 66–72
58. Schersten, B. and Fritz, H. (1967). Subnormal levels of glucose in the urine: a sign of urinary tract infection. *J. Am. Assoc. Physicians*, **201,** 949–952
59. Simmons, L.A. and Williams, J.D. (1962). A simple test for significant bacteriuria. *Lancet*, **1,** 1377–1378
60. Ampel, N.M. and Zinner, S.H. (1983). Bacterial urinary tract infection in pregnancy. In Francois, B. and Perrin, P. (eds.) *Urinary Infection: Insights and prospects*, pp. 141–160. (London: Butterworth)
61. Little, P.J. (1966). The incidence of urinary infection in 5000 pregnant women. *Lancet*, **2,** 925–928
62. Kincaid Smith, P. and Bullen, M. (1965). Bacteriuria in pregnancy. *Lancet*, **1,** 395–399
63. Kass, E.H. (1960). Bacteriuria and pyelonephritis of pregnancy. *Arch. Intern. Med.*, **105,** 194–198
64. Wilson, J.M.G. and Jungner, G. (1968). *Principles and Practices of Screening for Disease.* (Geneva: WHO)
65. Campbell-Brown, M., McFadyen, I.R., Seal, D.V. and Stevenson, M.L. (1987). Is screening for bacteriuria in pregnancy worthwhile? *Br. Med. J.*, **294,** 1579–1582
66. Le Blanc, A. and McGanity, W.J. (1965). A survey of bacteriuria in pregnancy. In Kass, E.H. (ed.) *Progress in Pyelonephritis*, pp. 58–63. (Philadelphia: F.A. Davis and Co.).
67. Naeye, R.L. (1979). Causes of the excessive rates of perinatal mortality and prematurity in pregnancies complicated by maternal urinary tract infection. *N. Engl. J. Med.*, **300,** 819–823
68. Sever, J.L., Ellenberg, J.H. and Edmonds, D. (1978). Urinary tract infections during pregnancy: Maternal and paediatric findings. In Kass, D.H. and Brumfitt, W. (eds.) *Infections of the Urinary Tract*, pp. 19–21. (Chicago: University of Chicago Press)

69. Kaitz, A.L. and Hodder, E.W. (1961). Bacteriuria and pyelonephritis of pregnancy: A prospective study of 616 pregnant women. *N. Engl. J. Med.*, **265**, 667–672
70. Turck, M., Goeffe, B.S. and Petersdorf, R.G. (1962). Bacteriuria of pregnancy. *N. Engl. J. Med.*, **266**, 857–860
71. McFadyen, I.R., Eykyn, S.J., Gardner, N.H.V., Vamier, T.M., Bennett, A.E., Mayo, M.E. and Lloyd-Davies, R.W. (1973). Bacteriuria in pregnancy. *J. Obstet. Gynaecol. Br. Commonw.*, **80**, 385–405
72. Sussman, M., Asscher, A.W., Waters, W.E., Evans, J.A.S., Campbell, H., Evans, K.T. and Williams, J.E. (1969). Asymptomatic significant bacteriuria in the non-pregnant woman. *Br. Med. J.*, **1**, 799–803
73. Kunin, C.M. and McCormack, R.C. (1968). An epidemiological study of bacteriuria and blood pressure among nuns and working women. *N. Engl. J. Med.*, **278**, 635–642
74. Kunin, C.M., Zacha, E. and Paquin, A.J. Jr. (1962). Urinary tract infections in school children: prevalence of bacteriuria and associated urological findings. *N. Engl. J. Med.*, **226**, 1287–1296
75. Verrier Jones, K., Asscher, A.W. and Verrier Jones, E.R. (1984). Long term aspects of covert bacteriuria: a 10 year follow-up of Cardiff schoolgirls. In Brodehl, J. and Ehrich, J.H.H. (eds.) *Paediatric Nephrology*, pp. 302–305. (Berlin: Springer Verlag)
76. Williams, J.D. (1984). Bacteriuria in pregnancy. In Asscher, A.W. and Brumfitt, W. (eds.) *Microbial Disease in Nephrology*, pp. 159–181. (Chichester: John Wiley and Sons)
77. Stuart, K.L., Cummins, M.B. and Chin, W.A. (1965). Bacteriuria, pre-eclamptic toxaemia and prematurity. In Kass, E.H. (ed.) *Progress in Pyelonephritis*, pp. 45–49. (Philadelphia: Davis and Co.)
78. Whalley, P.J. (1965). Bacteriuria in pregnancy. In Kass, E.H. (ed.) *Progress in Pyelonephritis*, pp. 51–57. (Philadelphia: F.A. Davis and Co.)
79. Savage, W.L., Hajj, S.N. and Kass, E.H. (1967). *Medicine* (*Baltimore*), **46**, 385–407
80. Layton, R. (1964). Infection of the urinary tract in pregnancy: An investigation of a new routine in antenatal care. *J. Obstet. Gynaecol. Br. Commonw.*, **71**, 927–933
81. Turner, G.C. (1961). Bacilluria in pregnancy. *Lancet*, **2**, 1062–1064
82. Sleigh, J.D., Robertson, J.G. and Isdale, M.H. (1964). Asymptomatic bacteriuria in pregnancy. *J. Obstet. Gynaecol. Br. Commonw.*, **71**, 74–81
83. Williams, J.D., Brumfitt, W., Leigh, D.A. and Precival, A. (1965). Eradication of bacteriuria in pregnancy by a short course of chemotherapy. *Lancet*, **1**, 831–834
84. Patrick, M.J. (1967). Renal infection in pregnancy II: Bacteriuria in pregnancy related to maternal factors. *Obstet. Gynaecol. Br. Commonw.*, **74**, 17–23
85. Williams, G.L., Campbell, H. and Davies, K.J. (1969). The influence of age parity and social class on the incidence of asymptomatic bacteriuria in pregnancy. *J. Obstet. Gynaecol. Br. Commonw.*, **76**, 229–239
86. Henderson, M., Entwistle, G. and Tayback, M (1962). Bacteriuria and pregnancy outcomes: Preliminary findings. *Am. J. Public Health*, **52**, 1887–1892
87. Monto, A.S. and Rantz, L.A. (1963). The development and character of bacteriuria in pregnancy. *Ann. Intern. Med.*, **59**, 186–193

88. Maskell, R. (1982). *Urinary Tract Infection.* (London: Edward Arnold)
89. Maskell, R. (1974). Importance of coagulase negative staphylococci as pathogens in the urinary tract. *Lancet,* **1,** 1155–1158
90. Meijers-Sever, G.J., Arnoudse, J.D., Mensink, W.F.A. and Dankert, J. (1979). The presence of antibody coated anaerobic bacteria in asymptomatic bacteriuria during pregnancy. *J. Infect. Dis.,* **140,** 653–658
91. McDowall, D.R.M., Buchanan, J.D., Fairley, K.F. and Gilberts, G.L. (1981). Anaerobic and other fastidious organisms in asymptomatic bacteriuria in pregnant women. *J. Infect. Dis.,* **144,** 114–122
92. Savage, J.A., Gilbert, G.L., Fairley, K.F. and McDowell, D.R. (1983). Bacteriuria due to *Ureaplasma urealyticum* and *Gardnerella vaginalis* in women with pre-eclampsis. *J. Infect. Dis.,* **148,** 605–606
93. Williams, G.L., Davies, D.K.L., Evans, K.T. and Williams, J.E. (1968). Vesicoureteric reflux in patients with bacteriuria in pregnancy. *Lancet,* **2,** 1202–1205
94. McLachlan, M.S.F., Meller, S.T., Verrier Jones, E.R., Asscher, A.W., Fletcher, E.W.L., Mayon-White, R.T., Ledingham, J.G.G., Smith, J.C. and Johnston, H.H. (1975). Urinary tract in schoolgirls with covert bacteriuria. *Arch. Dis. Child.,* **50,** 253–258
95. Kass, E.H. (1959). Bacteriuria and pyelonephritis of pregnancy. *Trans. Assoc. Am. Physicians,* **72,** 257–264
96. Whalley, P.J., Pritchard, J.A. and Richards, J.A. (1963). Sickle cell trait and pregnancy. *J. Am. Med. Assoc.,* **186,** 1132–1135
97. Giles, C., and Brown, J.A.H. (1962). Urinary infection and anaemia in pregnancy. *Br. Med. J.,* **2,** 10–13
98. Condie, A.P., Williams, J.D., Reeves, D.S. and Brumfitt, W. (1968). Complications of bacteriuria in pregnancy. In O'Grady, F. and Brumfitt, W. (eds.) *Urinary Tract Infection,* pp. 148–159. (London: Oxford University Press)
99. Stuart, K.L., Cummins, G.T.M. and Chin, W.A. (1965). Bacteriuria prematurity and the hypertensive disorders of pregnancy. *Br. Med. J.,* **1,** 554–556
100. Norden, C.W. and Kilpatrick, W.H. (1965). Bacteriuria of pregnancy. In Kass, E.H. (ed.) *Progress in Pyelonephritis,* pp. 64–72. (Philadephia: F.A. Davis and Co.)
101. Bryant, R.E., Windom, R.E. and Vineyard, J.P. Jr. (1964). Asymptomatic bacteriuria in pregnancy and its asociation with prematurity. *J. Lab. Clin. Med.,* **63,** 224–231
102. Low, J.A., Johnston, E.E., McBride, R.C. and Tuffnell, P.G. (1964). The significance of asymptomatic bacteriuria in the normal obstetric patient. *Am. J. Obstet. Gynecol.,* **90,** 897–906
103. Williams, J.D., Reeves, D.S., Brumfitt, W. and Condie, A.P. (1973). The effects of bacteriuria in pregnancy on maternal health. In Brumfitt, W. and Asscher, A.W. (eds.) *Urinary Tract Infection,* pp. 103–107. (London: Oxford University Press)
104. Ihle, B.U., Long, P. and Oats, J. (1987). Early onset preeclampsia: recognition of underlying renal disease. *Br. Med. J.,* **294,** 79–81
105. Sacks, S., Verrier Jones, K., Roberts, R., Ledingham, J.G.G. and Asscher, A.W. (1987). Outcome of pregnancy in women with childhood bacteriuria. *Lancet,* **2,** 991–994
106. Norden, D.W. and Tuttle, E.P. (1965). Impairment of urinary concentrating

ability in pregnant women with asymptomatic bacteriuria. In Kass, E.H. (ed.) *Progress in Pyelonephritis*, pp. 73–80. (Philadelphia: F.A. Davis and Co.)

107. Elder, H.A. and Kass, E.H. (1965). Renal function in bacteriuria of pregnancy: Its relationship to prematurity, acute pyelonephritis and excessive weight gain. In Kass, E.H. (ed.) *Progress in Pyelonephritis*, pp. 81–86. (Philadelphia: F.A. Davis and Co.)
108. Williams, G. (1969). Urine concentrating ability in women with asymptomatic bacteriuria in pregnancy. *Br. Med. J.*, **3,** 212–215
109. Harris, R.E. (1976). Infections of the urinary tract during pregnancy: Use of fluorescent antibody technique as an aid in patient evaluation. *South. Med. J.*, **69,** 1429–1432
110. Davison, J.M., Sprott, M.S. and Selkon, J.B. (1984). The effect of covert bacteriuria in schoolgirls on renal function at 18 years and during pregnancy. *Lancet,* **2,** 651–656
111. Leading article (1982). Kasstigating Kass. *Lancet,* **2,** 694–695
112. Stamm, W.E., Counts, G.W., Running, K.R., Fihn, S., Turck, M. and Holmes, K.K. (1982). Diagnosis of coliform infection in acutely dysiuric women. *N. Engl. J. Med.,* **307,** 463–468
113. Bollgren, I., Engstrom, C.F., Hammarlind, M., Kallenius, G., Ringertz, H. and Svenson, S.B. (1984). Low urinary counts of P fimbriated *Escherichia Coli* in presumed acute pyelonephritis. *Arch. Dis. Child.,* **59,** 102–106
114. Fairley, K.F., Bond, A.G., Brown, R.B. and Habersberger, P. (1967). Simple test to determine the site of urinary tract infection. *Lancet,* **2,** 427–428
115. Winberg, J. (1959). Renal functional studies in infants and children with acute nonobstructive urinary tract infections. *Acta Paediatr. Scand.,* **48,** 577–589
116. Stamm, W.E. (1983). Localisation of urinary tract infections. In Francois, P. and Perrin, P. (eds.) *Urinary Infection: Insights and Prospects,* pp. 47–71. (London: Butterworth)
117. Stamm, W.E., Wagner, K.F. and Amsel, R. (1980). Causes of the acute urethral syndrome in women. *N. Engl. J. Med.,* **303,** 409–415
118. Medical Research Council Bacteriuria Committee (1979). Recommended terminology of urinary tract infection. *Br. Med. J.,* **2,** 717–719
119. Egwnata, V.E. (1984). Spontaneous intraperitoneal rupture of pyelonephrosis during pregnancy. *Br. J. Urol.,* **56,** 224–225
120. Rubin (1987). *Prescribing in Pregnancy.* (London: British Medical Journal)
121. Wise, R. (1987). Prescribing in pregnancy: Antibiotics. *Br. Med. J.,* **294,** 1415–1417
122. Harris, R.E. and Gilstrap, L.C. (1974). Prevention of recurrence of pyelonephritis during pregnancy. *Obstet. Gynecol.,* **44,** 637–641
123. Bailey, R.R. (1983). *Single Dose Therapy of Urinary Tract Infection.* (Sydney: ADIS Health Science Press)
124. Conway, N. and Brit, B.D. (1965). Streptomycin in pregnancy: Effect on the foetal ear. *Br. Med. J.,* **2,** 260–263
125. Gruneberg, R.N., Leigh, D.A. and Brumfitt, W. (1969). Relationship of bacteriuria in pregnancy to acute pyelonephritis prematurity and foetal mortality. *Lancet,* **2,** 1–3
126. Naeye, R.L., Harkness, W.L. and Utts, J. (1977). Abruptio placentae and perinatal death: a prospective study. *Am. J. Obstet. Gynecol.,* **128,** 740–746

127. McGrady, G.A., Daling, J.R. and Peterson, D.R. (1985). Maternal urinary tract infection and adverse foetal outcome. *Am. J. Epidemiol.*, **121,** 377–381
128. Patrick, M.J. (1967). Influence of maternal renal infection on the foetus and infant. *Arch. Dis. Child.*, **42,** 208–213
129. Ives, J.A., Abbott, G.D. and Bailey, R.R. (1971). Bacteriuria in pregnancy and infection in amniotic fluid and infant. *Arch. Dis. Child.*, **46,** 82–84
130. British Medical Association and the Pharmaceutical Society of Great Britain (1987). *British National Formulary,* **13,** 263
131. Holland, N.H., Kotchen, T. and Bhathena, D. (1975). Hypertension in children with chronic pyelonephritis. *Kidney Int.*, **8,** S-243–251
132. Weinberger, M.H. and Weir, R.J. (1983). Oral contraceptives and hypertension. In Robertson, J.I.S. (ed.) *Handbook for Hypertension, Vol. 2. Clinical Aspect of Secondary Hypertension*, pp. 196–206. (Amsterdam: Elsevier Science Publications BV)
133. Bailey, R.R., Janus, E., McLoughlin, K., Lynn, K.L. and Abbott, G.D. Familial and genetic data in reflux nephropathy. In Hodson, J.H., Heptinstall, R. and Winberg, J. (eds.) *Reflux Nephropathy Update.* pp. 40–51. (Basel: Karger)
134. Gillenwater, J.Y., Harrison, R.B. and Kunin, C.M. (1979). Natural history of bacteriuria in schoolgirls – a long term case control study. *N. Engl. J. Med.*, **301,** 396–399
135. Smellie, J.M., Katz, G. and Gruneberg, R.N. (1978). Controlled trial of prophylactic treatment in childhood urinary tract infection. *Lancet,* **2,** 175–178

2

CHRONIC RENAL FAILURE

C. P. SWAINSON

INTRODUCTION

Women with renal disease worry, naturally, about their own abilities to conceive and bear a healthy child, and about the effects of such a pregnancy on their own renal disease. The answers they receive from their doctors vary a good deal and, until recently, have been relatively pessimistic. This reflects the medical profession's own uncertainties about the effects of pregnancy on the natural history of specific renal diseases. Doctors have generally erred on the side of caution and advised against pregnancy or recommended early abortion. There have been two major obstacles to further progress. The first is that most of the literature consists of small series of heterogeneous patients studied retrospectively and with rather short follow up. A second reason is poor documentation of the renal lesion and of the extent of renal dysfunction immediately prior to conception or early in the pregnancy. Work in the past 5–10 years has clarified some of these issues.

In general, if kidney disease progresses and renal function declines, woman's ability to sustain a viable pregnancy also decreases. Women with chronic renal disease, but with normal renal function (plasma creatinine $< 120\,\mu$mol/L) and who are normotensive, can expect to have a healthy pregnancy with a viable baby[1,2]. The natural course of their renal disease should be unaffected. These general statements should be modified for those women whose renal disease may follow an ominous course, for example adult polycystic kidney disease, focal glomerulosclerosis and, perhaps, IgA nephropathy. The prognosis for both mother and child is appreciably worse when renal function is definitely impaired prior to pregnancy or when the blood pressure is raised[1,3]. This is the difficult area for the clinician. Pregnancy in some patients will be quite uneventful; others will experience a severe decline in renal function which may not improve after delivery. Serious complications for the child, as well as the mother may occur. Women with advanced renal failure (blood urea >15 mmol/L; creatinine $>300\,\mu$mol/L) are not only unlikely to conceive but will have great difficulty in maintaining a normal gestation beyond the first trimester. Exceptions, however, do occur and some women have successfully borne healthy children while undergoing chronic ambulatory peritoneal dialysis or maintenance haemodialysis.

There will be those who disagree with a more optimistic prognosis but careful evaluation of the published data suggests that the above position is reasonable and that the prognosis for successful pregnancy in renal disease may vary across the world.

DETECTION OF RENAL FAILURE IN PREGNANCY

It is clearly important to establish the presence of renal disease early in pregnancy. The cardinal features to be looked for are: haematuria, proteinuria and *inappropriately low* renal function. A possible method of screening for renal disease is summarized in Table 2.1.

Proteinuria can be detected by commercially available test sticks. Any positive result should be checked with a 24 h urinary protein concentration. Proteinuria may increase during normal pregnancy from <150 mg/24 h to 300–500 mg/24 h. Gravid women are of an age when postural proteinuria may occur and this might only be detected during the gestation. Postural proteinuria is more common nearer term because of compression of the renal veins by the enlarged uterus and because women tend to assume a more lordotic posture.

Proteinuria may increase markedly in pregnant women with underlying renal disease, and, in the series of Katz *et al.*[1], was >3 g/24 h in 39 of 57 proteinuric women, some of whom developed the nephrotic

TABLE 2.1 Diagnosis of chronic renal disease

	Test	*Normal result*
Proteinuria	Dipstick	$-/+$: if $>+$, check 24 h urinary protein
Haematuria	Dipstick	$-$ve: if $+$ve, check microscopy
Blood pressure	Sitting quietly	$<130/80$ in weeks 1–24
Renal function	Plasma creatinine	<0.10 mmol/L or 1.1 mg/dl
	24 h creatinine clearance	>120 ml/min

syndrome. Heavy proteinuria may appear for the first time during gestation. The degree of proteinuria was generally well tolerated and had little effect on the subsequent course of renal disease or on fetal growth[1].

Haematuria

Haematuria remains a valuable screening test early in pregnancy. There is no evidence that excretion of red blood cells increases in normal women during pregnancy, and, therefore, the detection of significant haematuria (>10 rbc/ml) indicates possible renal disease. The finding of red cell casts is conclusive. Phase contrast microscopy of red cells in urine may disclose a large number of highly abnormal cells. When $>85\%$ of cells in haematuric non-pregnant women are abnormal, glomerulonephritis is likely; there is, however, no precise data in pregnancy.

Hypertension

Hypertension may be another useful sign of renal disease. In normal pregnancies, blood pressure decreases during the first and second trimesters, so that any woman presenting with a blood pressure > 130/80 mmHg in the first trimester of pregnancy should be regarded with suspicion. If further investigation fails to reveal renal disease, then it is likely she has essential hypertension or pre-eclampsia. Only 5% of pregnant women with hypertension have underlying renal disease[3].

Renal function

Failure to increase renal function early in pregnancy is a reliable guide to the presence of underlying chronic renal failure. Just as in non-pregnant women, alterations in the plasma creatinine concentration reflect changes in GFR. Mean values of plasma urea and creatinine concentrations in early normal pregnancy fall to 3.0 (20 mg/dl) and 0·05 mmol/L (0.6 mg/dl) respectively. The clearance of endogenous creatinine is a reasonable approximation of the glomerular filtration rate (GFR). Creatinine clearance is significantly elevated within four weeks of conception and reaches a maximal value of 40–50% above non-pregnant levels by 10 weeks in subjects without renal disease. An approximation, such as the nomogram by Cockcroft and Gault which requires only a knowledge of the patient's age, plasma creatinine and weight, is useful and as accurate as an out-patient 24-hour urine collection (Figure 2.1). Data in patients with chronic renal disease is sparse. Definite increments in GFR do occur early in the first trimester and are sustained throughout pregnancy in subjects with mild renal disease whereas no increase in GFR may occur in patients[4] whose plasma creatinine exceeds 123 μmol/L. Normal increments in haemodynamics have been demonstrated during pregnancy in transplant recipients who have good graft function.

$$\text{Creatinine clearance (ml/min)} = \frac{(140 - \text{age}) \times \text{weight (kg)}}{814 \times \text{plasma creatinine (mmol/L)}} \; [\times 0.85 \text{ for females}]$$

FIGURE 2.1 Cockcroft and Gault nomogram. When plasma creatinine is in mg/dl, the constant is 72 instead of 814

THE EFFECTS OF EXISTING RENAL DISEASE ON PREGNANCY

Two important determinants of successful pregnancy in women with renal disease are blood pressure and the level of renal function prior to pregnancy. It is difficult to assess the effect of pregnancy on blood pressure in women with renal disease. Katz et al.[1] studied 89 women with good renal function prior to conception and found significant hypertension occurred in 23%. Blood pressure had been elevated (>140/90 mmHg) prior to pregnancy in half of these cases. The rise in blood pressure was usually seen in the third trimester so that it was difficult to distinguish between superimposed pre-eclampsia and the effects of underlying renal disease. In some studies, hypertension has been observed to develop for the first time or become more marked. This occurred in a minority of pregnancies where the prepregnancy creatinine clearance was >80 ml/min.

The development of hypertension is associated with a higher perinatal mortality compared with normotensive pregnancies in women with chronic renal disease[1,5]. The presence of hypertension early in pregnancy or developing during the first trimester is therefore an ominous sign, especially if combined with an *inappropriately high* plasma creatinine concentration (i.e. one which has shown no reduction compared with prepregnancy values).

The plasma creatinine in the series of Katz et al. was <124 μmol/L and only 24 of 89 patients had proteinuria before pregnancy. Even in this group of women with relatively mild renal impairment, delivery occurred before 36 weeks in 20% of cases and a stillbirth rate of 5.7% was higher than that for all pregnancies at the centres studied. The neonatal death rate was 4.9% compared with 0.8% in the USA during the years studied (1956–1979). A detectable decrease in renal function occurred in 16% of these pregnancies and was reversed after delivery. Five patients developed end stage renal failure between 2 months and 8 years after delivery. In the view of the authors, pregnancy was thought not to have an adverse effect on maternal renal disease.

Data relating to perinatal mortality and maternal renal failure, closely related to pregnancy[3–5] is shown in Table 2.2. It is clear that there is a significant increase in perinatal mortality when the plasma creatinine is elevated in early pregnancy, but the effect on maternal renal disease is much less certain. When more serious renal failure is present, pregnancy may accelerate the decline in renal function. On the basis of rather sparse data, it is difficult to give a prognosis for an individual patient and there is little data published covering the past 8 years when there have been great advances in antenatal monitoring and neonatal care. In patients with renal disease, if the creatinine clearance increases during the first trimester by more than 25% and hypertension is not present, then a good outcome for both mother and child would be expected. If creatinine clearance fails to improve or worsens during the first trimester and significant hypertension appears for the first time, then a poor outcome for both mother and child seems likely. In between these two extremes, the present data does not allow more specific predictions.

In most studies of patients with plasma creatinine >130 μmol/L, any decline in renal function may be due to: (1) natural history of the underlying renal disease; (2) the effects of associated hypertension

TABLE 2.2 Effect of renal failure on obstetric outcome

	Plasma creatinine <130 μmol/L (1.5 mg/dl)		*Plasma creatinine >130 μmol/L (1.5 mg/dl)*	
	Perinatal mortality	*Renal failure*	*Perinatal mortality*	*Renal failure*
Bear[5]	1/36	0/29	0/7	4/8
Katz *et al.*[1]	2/70	0/70	—	—
Hou *et al.*[4]	0/10	0/18	3/15	1/7

which may be severe in this group; or (3) the specific effects of pregnancy. In general, if a woman has lost 50% of her renal function or the plasma creatinine is $>200\,\mu$mol/L, the risk of perinatal death is high. An irreversible decline in the mother's renal function, which may even necessitate dialysis, may occur. More commonly, however, the decline in renal function during pregnancy tends to improve after delivery in the majority of women. It is not possible currently to predict the prognosis for an individual[2], as the present data do not allow a more specific prediction.

ENDOCRINE EFFECTS OF RENAL FAILURE

Female patients with chronic renal failure report disinterest in sexual activity as well as loss of orgasm. In patients with chronic renal failure not on dialysis, oligomenorrhoea or amenorrhoea is present in at least 80% of patients. After dialysis has started, menstruation returns in about 60% of premenopausal women but menstrual disorders are still common in at least half of these women. It is not known with any certainty whether their cycles are ovulatory. Much less information is available on sexual dysfunction in women on dialysis than in men.

In premenopausal women, basal plasma luteinizing hormone (LH) concentrations are normal or elevated. The follicle-stimulating hormone (FSH) response to LH-releasing hormone (LH-RH) is normal but the LH response is delayed. Normal or elevated levels of LH are eventually reached with continuing stimulation. Oestradiol and progesterone levels are generally normal but oestradiol levels may be low if hyperprolactinaemia is also present. Indirect measures of ovulation, e.g. basal body temperature or vaginal cytology, indicate absent or rare ovulation and the preovulatory peak of plasma LH and oestradiol is frequently absent, suggesting a hypothalamic cause for anovulation. Lack of a preovulatory LH–FSH surge indicates disturbed positive oestradiol feedback. As a result, there is no rise of progesterone in the second half of the menstrual cycle, so that hypermenorrhoea and dysfunctional bleeding are common.

In postmenopausal women, gonadotrophins are as high as in non-uraemic postmenopausal women, but the menopause may occur earlier in women with chronic renal failure. Postmenopausal symptoms are unusual despite marked oestrogen deficiency.

It is not surprising that fertility is markedly reduced in uraemic women. Very little information is available but limited data indicates that early abortion and fetal wastage are markedly increased. A small number of women have carried pregnancies to term while on dialysis but most of these women have had some residual renal function. Despite the maternal deficiencies in 1,25-dihydroxy-vitamin D_3 and erythropoietin, fetal development was normal in these pregnancies although prematurity was common. Careful blood pressure control and maintenance of predialysis blood urea below 15 mmol/L requires increased hours and frequency of dialysis[6]. Daily or alternate day dialysis has been suggested by some authors and heparin administration must be controlled by careful laboratory monitoring.

Renal transplantation often restores fertility in premenopausal women. At least 1500 pregnancies in women with renal transplantations have been reported but this is likely to be a marked underestimate. Although no good epidemiological data are available, it has been suggested there is an increase in multiple births among renal transplant recipients, which would be consistent with residual hypothalamic–pituitary dysfunction. Deterioration of renal function during pregnancy, proceeding to postpartum rejection of a renal transplant, has been reported but is probably rare. Serious rejection episodes have been reported in up to 10% of pregnant renal graft recipients, but this is probably not significantly different from non-pregnant transplant patients.

THERAPEUTIC CONSIDERATIONS

There is no established treatment for diminished fertility in patients with chronic renal failure who are not on dialysis. If a woman on dialysis is having trouble with menstrual bleeding in the second half of the cycle, high doses of progesterone can be administered orally, either in the second half of the cycle only or continuously, or by intermittent intramuscular depot injection. Hysterectomy is only occasionally required to control uterine bleeding.

Bromocriptine, which has been shown to cause the resumption of ovulatory cycles, may be prescribed in an attempt to restore fertility. Pulsatile administration of LH–RH agonists to restore fertility has not been reported. If a female dialysis patient becomes pregnant or wishes to become pregnant with bromocriptine treatment, the dialysis schedule must be altered to try to maintain a predialysis blood urea of $< 15\,\text{mmol/L}$.

Pregnancy in a transplant recipient should not be encouraged until the graft has shown stable function for at least one year[6]. At this stage, the dose of corticosteroids and other immunosuppressive agents will be stable and at a maintenance level. When significant proteinuria, hypertension or evidence of graft dysfunction are present, pregnancy should be strongly discouraged. The incidence of both spontaneous abortion and fetal prematurity is increased. Contraceptive advice to premenopausal transplant recipients is controversial. Some specialists advise low-dose oestrogen oral contraceptives, despite their potential to aggravate hypertension or increase the risk of thromboembolism. There is no report of experience with intrauterine devices, and, indeed, there is no systematic study of contraceptive practice in the literature.

Limited information is available in female patients on chronic ambulatory peritoneal dialysis (CAPD). In one study, 6 out of 7 female patients under 45 years had regular periods, although there is no information on whether these were ovulatory. Winchester *et al.*[7] described a higher incidence of ovulation in patients on CAPD and successful pregnancies on CAPD have been reported.

REFERENCES

1. Katz, A.I., Davison, J.M., Hayslett, J.P., *et al.* (1980). Pregnancy in women with renal disease. *Kidney Int.*, **18,** 192
2. Davison, J.M., Katz, A.I. and Lindheimer, M.D. (1985). Renal disorders during pregnancy. *Clin. Perinatol.*, **12,** 497
3. Adams, E.M. and Finlayson, A. (1961). Familial aspects of pre-eclampsia and hypertension in pregnancy. *Lancet*, **2,** 1375
4. Hou, S.H., Grossman, S.D. and Madias, N.E. (1985). Pregnancy in women with renal disease and moderate renal insufficiency. *Am. J. Med.*, **78,** 185
5. Bear, R.A. (1976). Pregnancy in women with renal disease; A study of 44 cases. *Obstet. Gynecol.*, **48,** 13

6. Registration Committee of the European Dialysis and Transplant Association. (1980). Successful pregnancies in women treated by dialysis and kidney transplantation. *Br. J. Obstet. Gynaecol.*, **87**, 839
7. Winchester, J.F., Foegh, M. and Klober Danz, N. (1985). Return of menstruation and improvement of sexual function as a result of CAPD. *Abstracts II International Symposium on Peritoneal Dialysis*, Berlin, p. 75

3

PREGNANCY IN DIALYSIS AND TRANSPLANT PATIENTS

H. A. LEE

Our department, over the past 15 years, has secured a fairly comprehensive experience of pregnancy in both dialysis and transplant patients. For instance, the oldest patient on haemodialysis, aged 44, successfully delivered a live baby[1], whilst the first successful pregnancy in a diabetic patient having chronic ambulatory peritoneal dialysis was published five years ago[2,3]. We are also the unit to report the first baby born to a mother receiving cyclosporin A as the only immunosuppressive agent[4]. On the other hand, I suspect our department has the dubious record of having the fastest conception after successful transplantation, namely 3 weeks!

The first report of pregnancy after transplantation in a living related donor recipient (identical twin) was in 1958, when a live child was born to a mother who had not been maintained on immunosuppressive drugs. In 1966, two more living related donor recipients delivered two further normal children by vaginal deliveries and both of these were maintained on conventional treatment. In 1967, the first successful pregnancy following a cadaveric renal transplant was reported, and, in 1979, Rudolph *et al.* reviewed 440 pregnancies in transplant patients where 221 had achieved term deliveries and 54 premature births with a net failure rate of 175 (39.8%)[5]. In 1984, Davison[6] reviewed 1068 pregnancies in 717 patients (these included some of those previously reviewed by Rudolph) and the overall conclusion was that about 1 in 50 women of childbearing age with a functioning graft would become pregnant. This is also confirmed in the largest series attributed to one unit (Penn, 1985)[7].

The first description of a successful pregnancy in a haemodialysis patient was reported in 1975[8] whilst the first successful pregnancy in a patient on chronic ambulatory peritoneal dialysis was reported in 1983 (Cattran and Benzie)[9].

THE PORTSMOUTH EXPERIENCE (Table 3.1)

We have had one successful pregnancy on haemodialysis and one on chronic ambulatory peritoneal dialysis. Twelve transplant patients (11 cadaveric donor recipients) have had a total of 17 pregnancies. There were eight single pregnancies and four patients had multiple pregnancies, three patients having had two and one patient three pregnancies. The 17 pregnancies resulted in 13 live births with a mean gestational period of 37.7 weeks (which compares favourably with the EDTA 1987 figure of 38.5 weeks)[10]. There were two abortions for unwanted children, one therapeutic abortion in a mother with two healthy children already, who had her own polycystic kidneys *in situ* and who had impaired graft function, and one intrauterine death at 29 weeks in a patient whose fetus had marked renal dysgenesis and oligoamnios. One spontaneous abortion occurred at 16 weeks. Both the spontaneous abortion and the intrauterine death occurred in patients receiving cyclosporin A although both patients were requiring concurrent treatment with hypotensive agents, including captopril.

As a matter of interest, at least 12 males have become fathers on our programme, one on CAPD, two on haemodialysis and nine post-renal transplantation.

The mean birthweight of babies in our series was 2.87 kg which compares favourably with the ETDA 1987 report of 2.5 kg. Hypertension existed early in pregnancy in 6 of our patients and pre-eclamptic toxaemia occurred in two of these women, both of whom delivered live babies. Another two patients, with controlled hypertension from the beginning of their pregnancies lost their babies at 16 weeks and 29 weeks respectively. Careful control of hypertension is essential and agents such as methyldopa or labetalol and metoprolol may prove valuable occurring early on in pregnancy.

Caesarian section was performed in four of our pregnancies though only one was for fetal distress. The remaining three were undertaken early on in our experience, when, perhaps, there was an unjustified fear of either uterine dystocia or cephalopelvic disproportion. In our series, six mothers were on cyclosporin A as their only immunosuppressant agent and two of these lost their babies at 16 and 29 weeks, respectively. Both were also receiving captopril.

GENERAL REPORTS

In the 1980 EDTA/ERA report[11], successful pregnancies were recorded in 275 transplanted and 35 dialysis patients, resulting in the birth of 142 males and 159 females (in 16, the sex had not been recorded). By 1982, the largest number of successful pregnancies had been born to UK treated patients. There appeared to be a slight increase in multiple pregnancies in transplant patients. At the EDTA/ERA meeting in Berlin in 1987[10], it was reported that 490 successful pregnancies had been recorded in the Registry, resulting in 500 live babies. These included 8 sets of twins and one set of triplets; 0.4% of mothers were being treated by CAPD at the time of delivery, 11% by haemodialysis and the remaining 88% had functioning transplant kidneys. Almost 70% of the mothers were aged between 21 and 32 years at the time of delivery, with a range from less than 21 to more than 40. Approximately 40% of deliveries took place between two and four years after transplantation, although pregnancies occurred during the first year and as late as 10–12 years following transplantation.

Before 1982, 25–28% of pregnancies in grafted patients ended in therapeutic abortion. The reasons given were (a) unwanted children, (b) unstable renal function, (c) hypertension, and (d) hereditary disease (polycystic renal disease, diabetes mellitus, etc.). What is quite staggering is that the EDTA Registry, in 1980[11], enquired about the provision of contraceptive advice to women on renal replacement therapy. Of 752 centres in Europe who responded, only 11% gave contraceptive advice to all women of childbearing age, whilst a further 46% counselled some of their patients. Clearly, this is a fault that needs to be rectified; otherwise a continuing high proportion of preg-

TABLE 3.1 Details of some Portsmouth female transplantees or on

Patient and age (y)	*Tx date*	*Gestation (weeks)*	*On hypotensives*	*Child born*	*Delivery*
D.L. 22	15.5.84	(i) 39 (ii) ≈39.5	No No	9.4.85 29.9.87	Forceps Normal
S.A. 21	6.11.81	39.5	No	8.3.83	Induced, normal
D.W. 27	1.2.81	(i) 38 (ii) 37	Yes Yes	2.8.82 21.9.87	Forceps, normal
L.G. 25	10.6.83	38	Yes	13.1.88	Induced
C.B. 21	20.11.85	36	No	28.11.86	Caesarian
J.P. 34	26.9.74	(i) 38 (ii) 40	No	29.10.75 29.3.77	Caesarian Caesarian
L.B. 27	9.6.73	32	Yes	7.11.75	Caesarian
A.W. 28	23.10.84	29 (IUD)	Yes	28.2.88	Still birth
S.P. 27	4.3.82	16	Yes	15.3.88	Spontaneou abortion
E.K.* 32	4.4.78	39	No	3.12.84	Normal
V.C.† 30	14.12.78	28	No	14.12.80	Spontaneou normal delivery
R.E. 44	on H.D. for $2\frac{1}{2}$y	34	No	—	Caesarian
P.T. 26	CAPD started at 22 wks	35	No	—	Caesarian

* Living related donor

† Patient not aware she was pregnant till 20 weeks. Poor renal function. Ser

All live births survived

dialysis and their pregnancies

Fetal			Immunosuppression or dialysis	Original diagnosis
Length	*Head circumference*	*Weight (kg)*		
52	34	3.3	Cyclosporin A	Chronic
58	36.5	4.5	Cyclosporin A	pyelonephritis
—	—	3.01	Cyclosporin A	Chronic pyelonephritis
50	35	3.1	Cyclosporin A	Glomerulonephritis
47	32	2.5	Cyclosporin A	
48	33	2.95	Conventional	Glomerulonephritis
—	—	1.91	Cyclosporin A	DLE
47.5	—	2.83	Conventional	Polycystic
52.5	—	3.66	Conventional	kidneys
—	—	0.95	Conventional	Interstitial nephropathy
—	—	—	Cyclosporin A	V–U reflux and pyelonephritis
—	—	—	Cyclosporin A	Glomerulonephritis
—	—	3.2	Conventional	Chronic pyelonephritis
—	—	1.1	Conventional	Glomerulonephritis
42.5	31.5	1.93	Haemodialysis	Glomerulonephritis
42.5	29.5	1.7	CAPD	Diabetic nephropathy

creatinine 250 μmol/L. Graft failed 18/12 later.

nancies in transplant women of childbearing age will end in abortion. There is general agreement that the mini pill is acceptable, whilst there is a reluctance to use intrauterine devices for fear of associated infection. The alternative of the male using condoms, of course, is acceptable.

Clearly, the question of hereditary disease deserves special attention. However, many mothers who had hereditary disease as their cause of renal failure, e.g. polycystic renal disease and Alport's syndrome, have elected to become pregnant. As modern medicine advances, the views of such parents should be respected.

RENAL FUNCTION DURING PREGNANCY

The question of so-called deteriorating renal function during pregnancy requires a degree of redefinition now that many mothers are receiving cyclosporin A as their only immunosuppressive agent. Many mothers will have proteinuria from the beginning of their pregnancy but this may represent no more than protein leak from their own original kidneys. Rudolph *et al.*, 1979[5], noted that 17% of 125 mothers experienced a deterioration in renal function during pregnancy. In five of our patients, the same phenomenon was noted and two lost their kidneys postpartum. There is a tendency for proteinuria to increase during pregnancy but, as far as can be ascertained from the literature, this has little significance. Thus, a patient may have between 1 and 2 g of proteinuria at the outset of pregnancy; this may increase to 2–4 g by the third trimester but without any detectable clinical effect. With the advent of cyclosporin A, some patients will begin their pregnancies with serum creatinine concentrations in the range of 150–200 μmol/L. Provided such patients have been known to have stable renal function, say, in the preceding 6 months, then this so-called elevated serum creatinine concentration is no reason for recommending therapeutic abortion. Hypertension *per se* is not a reason for recommending termination of pregnancy; modern hypotensive agents are available which have no serious side effects either on (a) the mother or (b) the developing fetus. ACE inhibitors should not be used[16].

When better contraceptive counselling is offered to all women of childbearing age early after successful renal transplantation, the abortion rate recorded after 1982 should decrease considerably. As mentioned above, one of our patients actually conceived within 1 month of transplantation, a course that deserves little recommendation.

There has been a general tendency amongst nephrologists looking after female transplantees of childbearing age to recommend they should wait 2 years before becoming pregnant, in the hope that such babies born after that time would have a higher birthweight. However, statistics do not support this argument. In the Portsmouth series, the majority of women conceived well within 24 months of transplantation, all except one having had cadaveric renal transplants, and yet the mean birthweight was no less, in fact slightly better, than the EDTA/ERA Registry report.

About 25% of all patients studied were on antihypertensive therapy at the beginning of pregnancy and there is a reported incidence of pre-eclampsia in some 30% of such patients compared with only 8% in healthy patients.

Preterm delivery (less than 37 weeks) has been reported to occur in some 52% of transplant patients (in 3 of our series). Pre-eclamptic toxaemia was the main reason in 32.4% of these. It should be noted that, in the general population, premature delivery is twice as common in those patients with chronic hypertension or developing pre-eclamptic toxaemia. The gestational period in haemodialysis patients is approximately 33.2 weeks, i.e. considerably less than in transplanted patients. This, no doubt, relates to the increased frequency of anaemia and less good control of uraemia in haemodialysis patients. Graft obstruction to delivery was feared in the early years of cadaveric renal transplantation but is seldom a problem; in one series of 440 patients, only 6 (1.4%) experienced obstruction due to the transplant kidney. Caesarian intervention was as high as 47% in 1978 but had fallen to 25% by 1984 as confidence increased and it was appreciated that the graft itself produces little interference with delivery.

CYCLOSPORIN A AND PREGNANCY[12]

35 patients receiving cyclosporin A as immunosuppressive treatment have had 36 pregnancies (5 from the Portsmouth unit). 28 patients were receiving cyclosporin A post-renal transplantation (one having

had a combined renal and pancreatic transplant), one post-heart transplantation, one post-bone marrow transplantation and 5 others for a variety of autoimmune diseases. 6 patients (16.7%) had abortions in the first or second trimester, whilst 29 patients, 80.6%, completed pregnancy and all had live babies. 10 patients (27.8%) developed hypertension, and, in 23 patients (63.9%) where the duration of pregnancy was known, the gestational period was 36.1 weeks (i.e. 11 were preterm). The birth weight of full-term neonates varied between 2370–3200 g. One baby died in the neonatal period and he was found to have an absent corpus callosum. In our own series, 6 patients have been managed by cyclosporin A, 3 having given birth to 2 babies, one to one baby, one having had a spontaneous abortion at 16 weeks and another a stillbirth at 29 weeks as a result of renal dysgenesis and oligo-amnios. It has been suggested that cyclosporin A may pass the placental barrier and cause intrauterine growth retardation, although the global experience does not support this. Furthermore, in one of the babies born to a mother on cyclosporin A alone, there was no evidence of any impaired immunocompetence as judged by the dose response curves to phytohaemagglutination and Con A stimulation; indeed, the baby showed a slightly increased response. A recent report[13] has suggested that cyclosporin A might cause growth retardation of the fetus as a result of placental transfer, but we cannot support that view point. What has been well established is that cyclosporin A does appear in the colostrum and breastmilk, and, therefore, breastfeeding in such mothers is not recommended[4]. There has been no evidence of increased infection rates in the neonates born to mothers on cyclosporin A.

SEXUAL FUNCTION

In male patients, loss of libido and impotence is recorded in approximately 50% of individuals with chronic renal failure and about 8% may improve after conventional dialysis. Nevertheless, it is important to note that impotence may persist in 22–42% after transplantation. In female patients, there is a 25–30% incidence of lack of libido and impotence during chronic renal failure with only a 6% improvement after dialysis[14].

Pregnancy occurs in about 1 in 50 patients of childbearing age with successful transplants but in only 1 in 200 female haemodialysis patients of similar age. By 1981, only 8 successfully completed pregnancies had been reported in haemodialysis patients. In the EDTA/ERA 1987 report, 54 patients on haemodialysis had completed successful pregnancies. The mean gestational period was less than 38 weeks in 17% of patients, compared with 10% in the normal population. Perhaps it is encouraging, though no cause for complacency, that neonatal deaths occurred in only 1.8% of 500 babies. Perhaps more importantly, congenital defects were not noted with any increased frequency in dialysis or transplant patients compared with the normal population.

PREGNANCY AND IMMUNOSUPPRESSION

Pregnancy is often described as an 'immunologically privileged state', but is the same true for the renal graft? Thus, the question has been posed as to whether or not, during pregnancy, immunosuppressive drugs should be reduced irrespective of renal function. Penn (1985)[7], like Rudolph (1979)[5], noted a deterioration in renal function in 7% of pregnancies recorded in his 39 patients. Most patients, by the time they conceive, will have stable renal function on baseline immunosuppression; there can be little justification for changing that immunosuppressive regimen simply because they are pregnant, particularly when it is noted there is no increased incidence of congenital malformation in the babies born to such mothers. Furthermore, a number of authors have noted that renal function may deteriorate rapidly after successful delivery even when the immunosuppressive regimen had not been changed. If immunosuppression is decreased during pregnancy, is there an increased risk of renal function deteriorating post delivery? Certainly, the worry about an increase in infection rate in the neonates born of mothers who are immunocompromised has not been supported in the literature.

Should mothers with compromised renal function post-transplantation become pregnant? It has been Penn's advice that they should be counselled against pregnancy, although, as previously indicated, mothers maintained on cyclosporin A may have stable renal function but with serum creatinine concentration in the range of 150–200 μmol/L. In such situations, I would not counsel (a) against pregnancy or (b) the termination of pregnancy should it arise. By the same token, there will be a number of mothers coming to pregnancy who have controlled hypertension. If, however, (a) hypertension is not successfully controlled, or (b) renal function deteriorates during pregnancy, termination of pregnancy may be considered. It is perhaps of interest that both mothers in our series who lost their babies early in pregnancy (spontaneous abortion at 16 weeks, intrauterine death at 29 weeks) were hypertensive and had serum creatinine concentrations in the range of 150–200 μmol/L.

PREGNANCY IN MOTHERS ON EITHER HAEMODIALYSIS OR CAPD

Clearly, the chances of such females becoming pregnant are much lower than in those with successful transplants. Nevertheless, over recent years, there have been an increasing number of reports of successful pregnancies in mothers on such replacement treatments for end-stage renal failure. When such women become pregnant, it is important that their metabolic environment is as carefully controlled as possible. Thus, for mothers on regular haemodialysis treatment, careful control of blood pressure is required and attention to their nutritional status, with very careful control of the blood urea concentration so that it is maintained in the range of 15–18 mmol/L[1]. Thus, for some haemodialysis patients, an increased number of haemodialysis hours per week will be required to achieve these optimal biochemical results.

Similarly, CAPD patients may require an increased number of daily exchanges, although the volume of individual exchanges may be reduced from the standard 2 L to maybe 1.5 or even 1 L exchanges. However, as clearly shown in our diabetic patient, careful CAPD management can result in a normal delivery and live infant.

RISKS TO THE MOTHERS[7]

In situ carcinoma of the uterus is fourteen times more common in immunosuppressed transplantees than normal women, whilst *in situ* carcinoma of the cervix is five times more common. Also, carcinoma of the vulva is more common though there is no evidence to suggest that carcinoma of the breast or ovary is increased. Such observations indicate that these mothers must be carefully monitored for many years post-transplantation. It is often stated that 'pregnant mothers bloom', but, at the same time, during the euphoria of a successful post-renal transplantation life, potential parents must be reminded that 'parenthood is much longer than pregnancy'. Therefore, careful counselling is required, not only about contraceptive advice, but about potential longevity.

RISKS TO THE FETUS

As mentioned above, premature delivery is common in both dialysis and transplanted mothers. In dialysis patients, this is related to poor control of uraemia and an increased incidence of anaemia; in transplanted women, prematurity may be related to hypertension and possibly, though not proven, to the immunosuppressive agents used. Adrenal suppression may be anticipated in children born to mothers on conventional immunosuppression and should be appropriately treated. There is no good evidence of increased infection rates in neonates born to immunocompromised mothers.

There have been reports of an increased incidence of respiratory distress syndrome (RDS) in premature neonates born to both dialysis and transplanted mothers. In some of these reports, mothers have been given increased steroid dosages prior to elective deliveries to help prevent RDS in their babies, though this has not been shown to be of any value – an observation which must raise doubts on the efficacy of steroids in the RDS of infants. It is gratifying to note from the literature there is not an increased incidence of teratogenecity in neonates born to immunosuppressed mothers or, for that matter, fathers. Although, in the animal field, it has been shown that rats given large doses of 6 mercaptopurine (the main metabolite of azathioprine) have smaller litters and their progeny may have a greater number of stillbirths, no such evidence is available clinically. In Penn's Colorado series, followed up for a period of 11 months to 15 years, no problems have thus far been recognized.

GENERAL COMMENTS

Careful contraceptive and general parenthood counselling should be given to both dialysis and post-transplant patients, particularly as many females in this group will be of childbearing age. It must now be recognized that the chances of a woman becoming pregnant post-transplantation are at least four times greater than when she was treated by haemodialysis. The high rate of therapeutic abortion in the early years can no longer be justified. All patients who do become pregnant must be carefully monitored. Haemodialysis and CAPD patients may require greater dialysis frequency to maintain optimal biochemical equilibrium and higher haemoglobin concentration. Such patients will require to be monitored more frequently, necessitating an increased frequency of out-patient visits. Their weight, haemoglobin, serum biochemistry (in particular, blood urea and serum creatinine) and blood pressure all require careful control.

The fact that a patient has a raised serum creatinine (in the range 150–200 μmol/L) is not a reason for recommending (a) against pregnancy or (b) termination of pregnancy. Likewise, modern hypotensive agents can be successfully used to control hypertension without adverse effects on the fetus. Now that cyclosporin A is being increasingly widely used, it should be recognized that the serum creatinine concentration in such mothers may be higher than in those formerly conventionally immunosuppressed.

The high rate of caesarian section noted in the early series is no longer warranted in light of modern experience. Indeed, in one large series, only 1.6% of 440 mothers required caesarian section for proven uterine dystocia. Of course, the accepted indications for caesarian section remain, such as fetal distress, inco-ordinate uterine action, maternal distress or other medical indications prejudicing further development of the baby, such as pre-eclampsia.

The question of proteinuria also needs to be carefully reassessed by obstetricians[15]. Many patients will have proteinuria from the beginning of pregnancy and this may increase, to a limited degree, during pregnancy but have no clinical significance. Indeed, I would recommend against routine measurement of proteinuria in such patients. The suggestion that mothers should not contemplate pregnancy until 2 years post-transplantation can no longer be upheld.

When a patient does have a successful pregnancy and a caesarian section is contemplated, careful consideration should be given as to whether or not tubal ligation should be undertaken at the same time. Though conventionally immunosuppressed mothers may breastfeed, those on cyclosporin A must not. Evidence for compromised immunocompetence in neonates born to immunosuppressed mothers has not been published thus far. Although there is no objective evidence of an increased rejection rate during pregnancy or immediately postpartum, there can be no justification for reducing doses of immunosuppressives during pregnancy.

The ability of tranplanted women of childbearing age who have previously had chronic renal failure to fulfil their own life cycle by having normal children represents a major advance in the quality of life given to patients with endstage renal failure.

REFERENCES

1. Sheriff, M.H.R., Hardman, M., Lamont, C.A.R., Shepherd, R. and Warren, D.J. (1978). Successful pregnancy in a 44 year old haemodialysis patient. *Br. J. Obstet. Gynaecol.*, **85**, 386–389
2. Kioko, E.M., Shaw, K.M., Clarke, A.D. and Warren, D.J. (1983). Successful pregnancy in a diabetic patient treated with continuous ambulatory peritoneal dialysis. *Diabetes Care*, **6**, 298–300
3. Lee, H.A. and Searle, M. (1985). Dialysis, pregnancy and transplantation in a diabetic – An illustrated case report. *Practical Diabetes*, **2**, 29–32
4. Lewis, G.J., Lamont, C.A.R., Lee, H.A. and Slapak, M. (1983). Successful pregnancy in a renal transplant recipient taking cyclosporin A. *Br. Med. J.*, **286**, 603
5. Rudolph, J.E., Schweitzer, R.T. and Bartus, S.A. (1979). Pregnancy in renal transplant patients: a review. *Transplantation*, **27**, 26–9
6. Davison, J.M. (1984). Pregnancy in renal transplant recipients: clinical perspectives. *Contrib. Nephrol.*, **37**, 170–178
7. Penn, I. (1985). Pregnancy following renal transplantation. In Andreucci, V.E.

(Ed.) *The Kidney in Pregnancy*, pp. 195–204. (Boston: Martinus Nijhoff Publishing)
8. Ackrill, P., Goodwin, F.J., Marsh, F.P., Stratton, D. and Wagman, H. (1975). Successful pregnancy in patients on regular dialysis. *Br. Med. J.*, **2,** 172–174
9. Cattran, D.C. and Benzie, R.J. (1983). Pregnancy in a CAPD patient. *Peritoneal Dialysis Bull.*, **3,** 13–15
10. Dykes, S. (1988). Successful pregnancies in women on renal replacement therapy. European Dialysis and Transplant Association. (Personal communication)
11. Registration Committee of the European Dialysis and Transplant Association (1980). Successful pregnancies in women treated by dialysis and kidney transplantation. *Br. J. Obstet. Gynaecol.*, **87,** 839–845
12. Magrath, S.M. (1987). Sandimmune (cyclosporin A) in pregnancy. Personal communication. Sandoz Ltd., Basle
13. Pickerell, M.D., Sawers, R. and Michael, J. (1988). Pregnancy after renal transplantation: severe intrauterine growth retardation during treatment with cyclosporin A. *Br. Med. J.*, **296,** 825
14. Challen, S., Wing, A.J., Broyer, M. and Rizzoni, G. (1985). Successful pregnancies in women on dialysis treatment and with a transplant. In Andreucci, V.E., (Ed.) *The Kidney in Pregnancy*, pp. 186–194. (Boston: Martinus Nijhoff Publishing)
15. Davison, J.M., Elliott, R.W., Kerr, D.N.S., Proud, G., Taylor, R.M.R., Ward, J.K. and Wilkinson, R. (1982). Effect of pregnancy on renal function in kidney transplant recipients. *Clin. Exp. Hypertens.*, **81,** 322–324
16 Kreft-Jais, C., Plouin, P.-F., Tchobroutsky, C. and Boutroy, J. (1988). Angiotensin-converting enzyme inhibitors during pregnancy: a survey of 22 patients given Captopril and 9 given Enalapril. *Br. J. Obstet. Gynaecol.*, **95,** 420–422

4

PREGNANCY AND DIABETIC NEPHROPATHY

D. W. M. PEARSON AND H. W. SUTHERLAND

INTRODUCTION

Successful pregnancy depends on the ability of maternal physiology to adjust to the demands of the feto-placental unit[1]. In women with diabetes mellitus (DM), however, multisystem functional and occasionally anatomical changes may accompany the metabolic abnormalities which characterize the condition[1,2]. Pregnancy in a woman with DM thus merits particular attention. The ultimate goal in any pregnant woman is to achieve a healthy baby who will integrate into an enduring family unit. Both husband and wife need to appreciate the problems associated with diabetic pregnancy and the implications of diabetic complications, such as nephropathy, on long-term lifestyle, health and survival. To achieve the goal of a successful pregnancy in a young woman with insulin-dependent diabetes mellitus (IDDM), especially if microvascular complications are present, the patient requires knowledge of the importance of prepregnancy and pregnancy glycaemic control, the skills and facilities to achieve such control, the outlook and lifestyle which will allow her to apply her knowledge and skills, and careful co-ordinated care by a team comprising an experienced obstetrician, physician and neonatologist. Motivation to achieve this outcome is normally very high and most diabetic women can be reassured about a successful outcome of pregnancy. Nevertheless, in a few, the advisability of pregnancy needs to be carefully considered.

Before the discovery of insulin and its introduction into clinical practice in the early 1920s, women surviving with diabetes mellitus were usually chronically malnourished and infertile. If they happened to conceive, the predisposition to ketoacidosis induced by the increased metabolic demands of pregnancy often resulted in maternal death. Insulin therapy returned fertility to such women, and, over the past sixty years, maternal morbidity has almost disappeared. In centres with a particular interest in diabetic pregnancy, even perinatal mortality (PNM) is now approaching that of the background population[1–4]. This reduced PNM reflects many advances in obstetric, medical and paediatric practice. Notwithstanding, in many centres, diabetic women with microvascular disease affecting the retina and kidneys have been strongly discouraged from having a pregnancy and first trimester therapeutic abortion is still recommended if nephropathy producing persistent proteinuria is present prior to pregnancy. The advisability of pregnancy in diabetic women and the practical aspects of management of diabetic pregnancy will be considered in this chapter.

The term diabetes mellitus simply implies chronic hyperglycaemia without specifying pathogenesis or related pathology. The type of diabetes and extent of any related pathology must be taken into account in the prediction of pregnancy-related problems.

CLASSIFICATION OF DIABETES MELLITUS IN THE REPRODUCTIVE YEARS[5]

During reproductive life, most women with established diabetes mellitus will have type I or insulin-dependent diabetes mellitus (IDDM) presenting classically in childhood or adolescence with the fairly rapid onset of thirst, frequency of micturition and weight loss. Ketonuria and predisposition to ketoacidosis result from insulin deficiency due to a progressive destruction of the β cells in the islets of Langerhans. Although the symptoms may have been present for only a short time at diagnosis, it is known that immunological abnormalities, such as islet cell antibodies, may have been present for many months or years prior to the clinical diagnosis[6]. The predisposition to IDDM is associated[7] with certain HLA tissue types, e.g. DR3 or DR4. Current evidence suggests that an insult by a virus[8], chemical agent[9] or both[10] initiates an immunological response in a susceptible individual, producing insulitis and progressive β cell failure and, eventually, clinical diabetes mellitus. An autoimmune pathogenesis of DM is supported by the detection of islet cell antibodies[11] and T cell abnormalities[12] at diagnosis. Additionally, there is a higher incidence of other autoimmune conditions, such as thyroid disorders or pernicious anaemia, in women with DM than in those without. The degree of residual β cell insulin secretion may be assessed by measurement of plasma C peptide. Continued endogenous insulin secretion may occur for a variable period after diagnosis and affect metabolic control favourably. Because the complications of DM relate predominantly to the duration of diabetes, women are encouraged to complete child bearing at an early age.

IDDM may present for the first time during pregnancy as pregnancy offers no protection against diabetes. Indeed, the reverse is true as the requirement for insulin secretion is increased; also, pregnant women are particularly vulnerable to infections, particularly in the renal tract, which may precipitate or exaggerate the symptoms of diabetes. Early recognition of such insulin-dependent women during pregnancy is crucially important to allow the introduction of appropriate replacement therapy.

The other common type of diabetes is type II or non-insulin-dependent diabetes mellitus (NIDDM)[5] which classically presents in middle-aged or elderly subjects but can appear in younger women with symptoms of several months duration. The thirst and polyuria, in the form of frequency of micturition and nocturia, may be less acute and other symptoms, such as pruritus vulvae, may predominate. 80% of such individuals are overweight at diagnosis and a positive family history is common. The condition is characterized by a relative but not absolute deficiency of insulin, resistance to the metabolic action of insulin with regard to carbohydrate metabolism and no ketonuria[13]. If a woman with type II DM is still in the reproductive age group, she requires advice about careful monitoring prior to and during pregnancy similar to that given to a woman with pre-existing type I DM. Women with type II DM will often be older and may have macrovascular disease. If angina pectoris or another feature of ischaemic heart disease is present, pregnancy should be strongly discouraged. Obesity, which increases insulin resistance, complicates management during pregnancy and a dietary plan to achieve sustained weight loss and ideal body weight is a major part of the pre-pregnancy care programme. In addition to these two common types of DM, a very small number of pregnant women with pre-existing DM have secondary DM, e.g. following a pancreatectomy.

The microvascular complications of DM have been reported in association with all types of DM and affect the nervous system, cardiovascular system, kidneys and retinae. The complications of DM are related to the duration of the condition and are likely to be linked to long-term metabolic control[14]. The incidence of IDDM is increasing in childhood[15] and many women reach adulthood with longstanding complicated DM. During pregnancy in such women, major emphasis is placed on the importance of maintaining a safe and physiological intrauterine environment for the developing fetus. The cornerstone of management is the maintenance of strict maternal glycaemic control. It is also important to consider the impact of the complications of DM on the physiology of pregnancy and the impact of pregnancy on existing diabetic complications during and after pregnancy[16]. The future health of the mother is of supreme importance to the health and welfare of her developing child and the well being of the entire family[16].

PREPREGNANCY

The years, months and weeks prior to conception have a major influence on the outcome of pregnancy in diabetic women and prepregnancy care should extend from the time of diagnosis[17,18]. The objective at this time should be to try to minimise the development of complications because women with longstanding diabetes mellitus complicated by microvascular changes are a high-risk obstetric group. The population requiring formal prepregnancy advice includes all fertile insulin-dependent diabetic women. Organization of diabetic services for young girls is necessary to review growth and development regularly, to make effective contraceptive advice available, to help children with diabetes make a successful transition to adulthood through the difficult adolescent years, to continue education and to identify, treat and slow the progression of diabetic complications. When pregnancy is contemplated or is manifest, appraisal of the renal functional status is essential and should be interpreted in the context of the following.

RENAL CHANGES IN PREGNANCY AND DIABETES MELLITUS

A spectrum of diabetes-induced renal changes ranges from almost normal renal function to endstage renal failure. Pregnancy can be superimposed at any stage of this continuum and it is necessary to consider how pregnancy may interact with such a variety of renal abnormalities.

Pregnancy

Some of the physiological adaptations to pregnancy[19] which occur in non-diabetic women are similar to those found just after the diagnosis of diabetes mellitus. In non-diabetic pregnancy, renal size is increased, partly due to an increase in glomerular size without an increase in cell number. Effective renal plasma flow (ERPF) and glomerular filtration rate (GFR) increase soon after conception. The mechanisms of the altered renal haemodynamics have not been clearly defined but may reflect a number of cardiovascular and endocrine changes. The increase in cardiac output produces a rise in effective renal plasma flow and thereby raises filtration pressure which will be enhanced by the decreased intraglomerular osmotic pressure associated with the physiological reduction of albumin concentration. The endocrine changes in pregnancy include enhanced production of aldosterone, deoxycorticosterone, progesterone, cortisol, human placental lactogen and human chorionic gonadotrophin, all of which may influence renal haemodynamics. Since the glomerular filtration rate increases without substantial alterations in the production of creatinine and urea, plasma levels of these solutes decrease even before the dilutional effect of the expanded extracellular volume takes place. Clinicians should be aware of the physiological changes occurring and that a urea concentration greater than 3.5 mmol/L and creatinine greater than 75 μmol/L may indicate underlying renal pathology, and, in pregnancy, posture may produce significant effects on the estimation of creatinine clearance.

Diabetes mellitus

Following the diagnosis of diabetes mellitus, there are several phases of altered renal function which relate principally to the duration of the condition. Other factors, such as glycaemic control, hypertension and protein intake, influence short-term renal function and also the progression to established renal failure which will occur in 30–40% of people with IDDM[20]. Two early changes of renal function which can be detected in IDDM are an increase in the glomerular filtration rate (GFR) and an increase in the urinary loss of albumin.

At the onset of DM, glomerular filtration rate is increased[21] by more than 40%. Reduction follows initial insulin therapy but correction of the hyperfiltration remains incomplete. During conditions of ordinary metabolic control on standard insulin therapy, GFR is elevated, for example, in non-proteinuric diabetic children and in young adults after 1–15 years of diabetes. This rise in GFR is induced by even moderate hyperglycaemia and by increases in glucoregulatory hormones, including glucagon[22] and growth hormone[23]. The increased GFR is associated with an increase in kidney size. Large kidneys mainly reflect an increase in tubular mass but large glomeruli are also present, indicating the surface area available for filtration. The increase in glomerular filtration rate is one of the factors predisposing to ultrafiltration in diabetic renal disease. Other factors thought to be important include renal plasma flow, transglomerular hydraulic pressure and the ultrafiltration coefficient which is a product of the water permeability of the glomerular capillary wall and the actual surface area available for filtration[21].

Another renal abnormality encountered in early diabetes is increased urinary excretion of albumin[24]. This is below the limit of detection by conventional urine tests for albumin (e.g. Albustix tests) but above the normal values of up to 20 mg albumin per 24 h. With the excretion of greater than 250 mg/24 h, the Albustix test becomes positive. The transition from normal, or near normal, protein excretion to overt nephropathy remains ill-defined. This subject is an area of intensive research because of its clinical importance, namely, during this transition stage, therapeutic intervention by control of hypertension, tight glycaemic control[25] or dietary modification may influence the progression from microalbuminuria to established proteinuria and irreversible renal damage[26].

The increased rate of albumin excretion is associated with an increase in blood pressure. Even this slight increase in blood pressure may influence the progression of nephropathy[26].

Established diabetic nephropathy is usually recognized clinically by the detection of Albustix-positive proteinuria which is initially intermittent, but subsequently persistent and is followed over a variable period by heavy proteinuria and a decline in glomerular filtration rate. The young person may be asymptomatic but histological changes in the glomeruli and blood vessels are well recognized. The glomeruli in diabetic nephropathy show a variety of histological features, including the classical nodular lesions described by Kimmelstiel and Wilson – diffuse intercapillary glomerulosclerosis, exudative or fibrin cap lesions and capsular drop lesions. The detailed mechanisms leading to such changes in DM are unclear. A retrospective analysis of more than 1400 autopsy specimens documented clearly a relationship between the increasing duration of diabetes and the presence of glomerulosclerosis[27]. On the basis of the evidence from human studies on renal-transplanted diabetic patients[28] and non-diabetic patients and animal studies[29], it appears that diabetic nephropathy is a consequence of the biochemical abnormalities associated with the disorder rather than the consequence of a separately inherited predisposition.

Diabetic nephropathy is characterized by a thickening of the capillary basement membrane of the glomerulus, alterations in the membrane chemical composition and changes in enzyme activities involved in its biosynthesis. The basement membranes from both normal and diabetic subjects are composed of glycoprotein- and collagen-like material containing substantial amounts of the aminoacids, hydroxyproline, hydroxyleucine, glycine and cystine, together with the sugars, galactose and glucose. The remainder of the carbohydrate is in the form of a heteropolysaccharide containing fructose, mannose, galactose, sialic acid and glucosamine. As with other glycoproteins, the synthesis of glomerular basement membrane probably occurs in several steps and the increased quantity of basement membrane glycoprotein demonstrated in diabetic nephropathy may have resulted from hyperglycaemia producing inappropriate or excessive glycosylation and thereby substantially altering the biochemical structure and function of the membrane. Estimation of glycosylation of haemoglobin has proved clinically useful[30] as an index of longer term diabetic control. Many body proteins, including lens crystallin[31], collagen[32], albumin[33] and lipoproteins[34], can, however, undergo post-translational modification by glycosylation and the function of these molecules may be affected by such structural alterations. The prospect of reversing functional deterioration by scrupulous metabolic control is an attractive notion prompted by the fact that microalbuminuria can be reduced by improved glycaemic control. The limits to which this can be achieved have still to be defined.

CLINICAL ASPECTS OF PREPREGNANCY CARE

When a woman with DM contemplates child bearing, formal prepregnancy assessment and advice should be available from an obstetrician and physician with a complementary interest in diabetic pregnancy. When the decision is taken to attend for prepregnancy counselling, the advisability of pregnancy and optimal timing of conception must be carefully considered. When diabetic nephropathy is present, most authorities would not encourage pregnancy since, although the outlook for that pregnancy may be good if optimal metabolic control is achieved prior to and during pregnancy, long-term maternal health may be disadvantaged – although the availability of kidney transplant has moderated this view in recent years. Persistent proteinuria in insulin-dependent diabetes mellitus is associated with much higher relative risk of renal failure and/or cardiovascular disease[35] than if proteinuria is absent.

Although effective means of managing renal failure by chronic ambulatory peritoneal dialysis, haemodialysis and renal transplant therapy are available, implications of such therapeutic techniques for a mother with a young family should be anticipated. Successful pregnancy has been reported following renal transplantation but advanced diabetic vascular disease puts these pregnancies at significant risk. Ogburn and co-workers reviewed nine cases of pregnancy complicated by diabetes and prior renal transplantation[36]. Maternal and fetal death occurred in a patient with foot and leg ulcers, and pregnancy-induced hypertension occurred in six patients.

Having discussed all the relevant aspects with both partners, however, the decision to proceed with pregnancy still rests with the woman. It is important that contact with the prepregnancy clinic is not lost because the outcome can be significantly influenced by optimizing glycaemic control prior to conception.

Even in specialist referral centres, perinatal mortality in pregnancies complicated by diabetes is increased. This is largely attributable to the increased incidence of congenital malformations in the infants of diabetic mothers. Several studies, but particularly that of Fuhrmann *et al.*[17], have shown that the incidence of congenital malformations can be reduced to that of the background population by improving maternal glycaemia prior to, and at the time of, conception and during organogenesis. The steps taken at the prepregnancy clinics to optimize metabolic control include modification of diet, insulin therapy and insulin regimen on the basis of home blood glucose monitoring results. Glycosylated protein estimation will give a good index of longer term diabetic control. Careful clinical assessment of retinal and renal function is essential.

Although the majority of diabetic women attending for prepregnancy care will not have objective evidence of renal disease by Albustix testing, microalbuminuria may be present[24]. Assessment of renal function by creatinine clearance estimation and 24 h urinary protein excretion provides useful baseline information prior to pregnancy. It is particularly important to detect and treat occult urinary infection in diabetic pregnancy because urine infection is a common reason for reduced metabolic control in diabetic pregnancy. It may also impair or lead to further diminution of renal function. One aspect of prepregnancy management must be counselling with regard to expectations of pregnancy and clinical management during the course of pregnancy. Women with significant renal disease should be advised that frequent hospital admissions may be required. Hypertension found before pregnancy should be controlled by β-blockers, hydralazine or α-methyldopa.

Delay in conception is indicated until any proliferative retinopathy has been fully treated by laser photocoagulation and blood pressure control has been optimized. Very rarely, macrovascular disease may be identified in older diabetic women and such women should be strongly advised against pregnancy. Successful pregnancy has been reported in a woman following coronary artery bypass grafting[37].

In addition to considering problems immediately related to diabetes mellitus and its complications, women should be counselled and assessed at the prepregnancy clinic on aspects of their general health, e.g. rubella immune status, cigarette and alcohol consumption, and drug therapy. Infertility can be identified and investigated. If ovulation is occurring, women are advised to use effective mechanical contraception until optimal resolution of clinical and social problems has been attained. The menstrual cycle can be characterized and ovulation identified by the use of several possible methods, e.g. urinary luteinizing hormone (LH surge), serum progesterone, ultrasound visualization or measurements of basal body temperature, so that conception may be accurately dated and delayed implantation identified. In women a complicated pregnancy, it is particularly important to establish gestational age accurately to determine the optimal time for delivery. Gestational age assessed by early ultrasound scanning may be misleading because of initial growth delay[38] which is itself more likely to occur if glycaemic control is poor and fetal malformation is manifest. If pregnancy is confirmed elsewhere, early referral to a specialist clinic is indicated. Women should be encouraged to attend for care as soon as pregnancy is suspected.

CLASSIFICATION OF DIABETES MELLITUS DURING PREGNANCY

As early as 1949, the duration of diabetes mellitus, age of onset and the presence of vascular disease were identified by Pricilla White as factors which have a prognostic value for pregnancy outcome. This led to the now widely used White's Classification[39] which has been extended to incorporate newer developments, *viz*:

Class A: managed by dietary therapy alone and would include gestational diabetes mellitus (GDM).

Class B: age of onset of diabetes mellitus 20 years or older and duration less than ten years.

Class C: onset age 10–19 years and duration 10–19 years.

Class D: onset age under 10 years, duration over 20 years, background retinopathy or hypertension (not pregnancy-induced hypertension or pre-eclampsia).

Class R: proliferative retinopathy or vitreous haemorrhage.

Class F: nephropathy with over 500 mg/day proteinuria.

Class RF: criteria for both classes R and F.

Class H: atherosclerotic heart disease clinically evident.

Class T: prior renal transplantation.

By definition, Classes A, B and C have no obvious vascular disease, but, in future, this may need to be reconsidered with the development of techniques to measure microalbuminuria. Class D refers to women with long duration of diabetes and also women with background diabetic retinopathy or hypertension at the beginning of pregnancy, irrespective of onset and duration of diabetes mellitus. Classes R, RF, H and T include women who have clinical evidence of significant vascular disease. Clearly White Class may change during pregnancy with the firm diagnosis of newly recognized complications. For the diagnosis of diabetic nephropathy in pregnancy, the cut-off figure of urinary protein excretion measured prior to the 20th week of pregnancy in the absence of urinary tract infection has varied in different reported series but usually is between 400–500 mg/24 h.

If abnormal carbohydrate metabolism is first detected during pregnancy, gestational DM (GDM) is diagnosed. Although, as noted above, a few symptomatic women may have spontaneous and/or latent type I DM precipitated by pregnancy, the majority of women with GDM have no symptoms of hyperglycaemia. They may, however, be identified by a variety of 'risk factors' or 'indicators', including glycosuria in a second fasting urine sample, previous heavy-for-dates or stillborn baby, a previous history of GDM or obstetric problems, such as hydramnios[1]. Such clinical indicators are neither sensitive nor specific. It has been suggested that a random, meal-related blood glucose sample should be taken as a screening test with a subsequent 75 g oral glucose tolerance test as the diagnostic procedure[40]. Another approach followed and recommended in the United States is that all women have a venous blood glucose estimation one hour after a 50 g oral glucose drink; a diagnostic 100 g oral glucose tolerance test (OGTT) may thereafter be used to identify GDM[41]. Pregnancies in women with GDM are identified as high risk and it should be appreciated that some may go on to develop diabetes in later life. However, patients in this group will not be considered further in this chapter.

EARLY PREGNANCY

The developing fetus and placenta are not autonomous but depend on maternal fuels and oxygen. The carefully controlled intrauterine environment depends on the flexibility of maternal metabolism during periods of feeding, fasting and exercise. As a corollary, early pregnancy hormones will influence maternal physiology which undergoes major changes during the early weeks of pregnancy. Cardiac output rises quickly in the first trimester to a level some 1.5 L/min above the non-pregnant level and this is maintained for the rest of pregnancy[19]. Arterial blood pressure may be relatively unaffected with a decrease in diastolic blood pressure in mid pregnancy. The unchanged blood pressure, despite the rise in cardiac output, is explained by a fall in peripheral resistance which reflects a tendency to peripheral vasodilatation during pregnancy. The mechanisms involved are not fully understood but include a marked resistance to the action of angiotensin, perhaps due to the effect of progesterone so that the pregnant woman is much more dependent on sympathetic tone to maintain blood pressure. During pregnancy, ganglion blocking drugs may produce a striking fall in blood pressure with changes in posture[19].

In practical terms, management of diabetes mellitus must allow for such changes in physiology. Insulin requirements may fall due to a decreased energy intake associated with loss of appetite. Hypoglycaemia and rebound hyperglycaemia may cause difficulties; family members should be instructed in the recognition and management of hypoglycaemia and have glucagon available for subcutaneous administration. In early pregnancy, a short hospital admission may be useful to review overall management and optimize the insulin regimen, particularly if women have not attended for prepregnancy counselling. There is often the need to change twice-daily insulin to multiple insulin injections, e.g. by separating the evening insulin to take soluble (fast-acting insulin) before the main evening meal and isophane (intermediate-acting insulin) before bedtime. Additional insulin may also be required before lunch to avoid late afternoon hyperglycaemia. The use of human insulins or highly purified porcine insulins is recommended during pregnancy since such insulins are less immunogenic and immunoglobulins are known to cross the placenta[42]. Frequent dietary assessment and advice is required to ensure an appropriate distribution of carbohydrate, fibre and an adequate energy intake.

Ultrasonic examination in mid-pregnancy provides help with the determination of gestational age and it may confirm the date of conception or initial growth delay suspected from earlier scans[38]. Congenital abnormality may also be recognized if present.

In women with long-standing diabetes and evidence suggesting underlying renal dysfunction, detailed clinical and biochemical assessment is necessary. While it is important that pre-existing proliferative retinopathy is identified and treated during the prepregnancy assessment, it is recognized that retinopathy can deteriorate during pregnancy despite optimal metabolic glycaemic control. Following careful study, Serup[43] emphasized that retinopathy which progresses during pregnancy often regresses in the puerperium and regular review by an experienced ophthalmologist is necessary. The pathophysiology of the progression of retinopathy during pregnancy and resolution postpartum is not clear. Regular detailed fundoscopy throughout pregnancy is particularly important in women with renal disease[44].

CLINICAL MANAGEMENT DURING PREGNANCY

At each visit, urine can be tested simply by diagnostic stick techniques for glucose, ketones and protein. The development of Albustix-positive proteinuria in the absence of urinary infection is significant and proteinuria should be quantified. More refined techniques have allowed the identification of quantities of albumin which were not detectable by Albustix. The presence of microalbuminuria may predict the outcome and so indicate appropriate management. Urinary excretion of albumin has been reported in non-diabetic women and the excretion rate was not found to be increased during pregnancy or to differ from that of a group of non-pregnant women[45]. In contrast, women with diabetes mellitus may show an increase in urinary albumin excretion during pregnancy. Although the White Classification separates diabetic women by the duration of diabetes mellitus and the presence of complications, future subclassifications may identify diabetic women with normal or increased albumin excretion during pregnancy if there is found to be prognostic value in this approach.

Hypertension in diabetic pregnancy

In women with diabetogenic microvascular disease, the development of significant hypertension during pregnancy is common[46,47]. Clinicians should try to differentiate chronic hypertension from pregnancy-induced hypertension (PIH) although both may be present. Diamond *et al.*[48] found that chronic hypertension was present in older women who usually did not have long-standing diabetes mellitus. In contrast, pregnancy-induced hypertension was more common in White Classes D, F and R (13/30 patients). Chronic hypertension should be diagnosed and treated prior to pregnancy and PIH may be reduced by prepregnancy counselling to optimize metabolic control. Jovanovic[49] has suggested that a blood pressure of less than 160/90 does not require specific therapy but β-blockade, hydralazine or α-methyldopa may be indicated if hypertension becomes more marked. Thiazide and loop diuretics should be avoided during pregnancy because maternal plasma volume expansion is an important maternal physiological adaptation. Nonetheless, fluid retention may become a problem, as will be discussed later.

If hypertension develops in pregnancy, glomerular filtration rate and effective plasma renal flow decrease by approximately 25% below predicted normal values. As these, however, are 30–50% above non-pregnant levels, both GFR and ERPF may remain elevated[19]. GFR decreases more than ERPF and therefore the filtration fraction diminishes. The ability to excrete sodium is usually impaired in the pre-eclamptic patient although pre-eclampsia can occur in the absence of fluid retention. Even when oedema is present, plasma volume is usually decreased in comparison with normal pregnancy[19]. Uric acid clearance also decreases and proteinuria is variable. Important factors in the development of proteinuria seem to be the haemodynamic determinants of GFR and the electrostatic properties of the glomerular wall. Reduced renal plasma flow, loss of the glomerular fixed negative charge and the presence of polyanions have been implicated in the pathogenesis of pre-eclampsia. The basement membrane biochemical changes associated with DM may explain the increased frequency of pre-eclampsia (PET) found in diabetic pregnancy. If proteinuria develops, the patient should be admitted to hospital for supervision of blood pressure, proteinuria and renal function.

Metabolic measurements

While the clinical team are concentrating on detailed biological and physiological assessments, the mother also has to carry out careful measurements.

In all women, the ability to measure blood glucose at home 4–6 times daily allows achievement of nearly normal blood glucose. It is important to provide a quality control on home blood glucose monitoring by comparing results with laboratory values or checking in-patient glucose profiles. If home glucose levels are raised, a test for urinary ketones must be performed. When ketonuria is detected, urgent admission is indicated since ketosis can develop rapidly during pregnancy and may be harmful to the fetus. The level of glycosylated haemoglobin will give an index of long-term diabetic control during pregnancy. In women with nephropathy, regular estimates of 24 h urinary protein excretion and creatinine clearance are important to quantify any deterioration in renal function.

The particular problems of pregnancy associated with diabetic nephropathy

Series of pregnant women with diabetic nephropathy have been reported by Kitzmiller *et al.*[50], Hare and White[51], Grenfell *et al.*[46],

Nesler *et al.*[47], Diamond *et al.*[48] and Dicker *et al.*[52]. The pregnancy experiences reported extend over many years and include data collected prior to the advent of modern methods of metabolic or fetal monitoring. Nevertheless, such clinical series give very useful descriptive clinical information on this relatively uncommon problem for many clinicians. From review of these reports, it appears that, in women with diabetic nephropathy, impaired creatinine clearance does not deteriorate during and after pregnancy more than would have been predicted without pregnancy. Proteinuria increases from the first to the third trimester and one of the factors which appeared to predict a poor perinatal outcome was proteinuria greater than 3 g/24 h in the first trimester or 10 g/24 h in the third trimester. Proteinuria and creatinine clearance returned to prepregnancy levels in the postnatal period and the striking increase in urinary albumin excretion in the presence of diabetic nephropathy presumably relates to the additional physiological adaptations of glomerular permeability during pregnancy. In most series, maternal hypertension was associated with proteinuria and correlated negatively with infant birthweight. Hypertension was treated by bed rest, methyldopa, β-blockers and hydralazine. Supine posture reduced cardiac output and renal plasma flow, and resting on the left lateral position to raise renal perfusion and thereby GFR was recommended. If the marked physiological expansion of the intravascular compartment in the presence of underlying diminished cardiac function leads to congestive cardiac failure, diuretic therapy is essential. Otherwise, diuretic therapy is to be avoided.

Modern obstetric and medical practice still depends on careful, regular clinical examination. Clinical or ultrasonic evidence of the development of polyhydramnios should be sought frequently because strict glycaemic control and bed rest are required to reduce or avoid the morbid consequences.

In addition to renal disease, many women had established retinopathy, and, in White's series, ten patients showed significant deterioration of diabetic retinopathy early in the course of gestation. The development of preretinal or vitreous haemorrhage resulted in the loss of vision in eleven of the twenty eyes. However, even in this series, 90% of the women showed no change in visual acuity.

Since that study was reported, laser therapy has become available to treat proliferative retinopathy. In many instances, the progression of diabetic retinopathy may be retarded in pregnancy by early and effective laser therapy. As noted above, Serup[43] has emphasized that many of the retinal changes spontaneously resolve after delivery and any decision about the need for laser therapy should be made by an experienced ophthalmologist. In all cases with nephropathy, regular retinal examination is mandatory with early referral for specialist ophthalmological assessment if preproliferative or proliferative changes develop. The presence of widespread microvascular disease may be mirrored in the placental changes in this group of women, namely decrease in size with excessive narrowing of vessel luminae, hyalinization and infarction. Impaired fetal growth is recognized in such pregnancies and presumably this relates to poor placental development and function with impaired oxygen and fuel transport. In contrast to infants of mothers with uncomplicated diabetes mellitus, infants of mothers with diabetic nephropathy are often small for gestational age. The macrosomia classically associated with diabetic pregnancy is presumed to relate to excessive availability of energy substrates, such as glucose, lipids and amino acids, from the maternal circulation. In response to these substrates, fetal β-cell hyperplasia occurs, producing hyperinsulinism and subsequent fetal adiposity and organomegaly[53,54].

Recognition of these problems associated with pregnancy in diabetic nephropathy promotes the development of appropriate clinical strategies. Regular clinical and ultrasonic assessment is required to diagnose intrauterine growth retardation. Careful monitoring of blood pressure, weight gain, renal and retinal status is essential. In the third trimester, fluid retention and hypertension may pose particular problems. At this stage, most patients with significant nephropathy are managed as inpatients with regular biophysical fetal assessment, including at least regular, frequent cardiotocography and detailed ultrasonography to identify the compromised fetus requiring early delivery. Kick charts are recorded on a daily basis by the patient and may provide a useful method of assessing fetal well-being.

Insulin requirement increases as pregnancy progresses, usually twofold. Women should be warned about this and know how to increase insulin and maintain normoglycaemia as pregnancy progresses. They should be reassured that their diabetes is no worse, only that this is to be expected in pregnancy. Throughout pregnancy, the need for effective communication between obstetrician, diabetic physician and neonatologist must continue, ideally in the setting of a multidisciplinary clinic with input from ophthalmologist and nephrologist as required.

DELIVERY

The timing of delivery in a diabetic woman depends on the progress during pregnancy, but, in an uncomplicated situation, many women deliver at term[2]. Diabetes mellitus alone is not an indication for caesarean section and the mode of delivery will be dictated by obstetric factors if normoglycaemia has been achieved. In a woman with diabetic nephropathy, early delivery may be precipitated by a number of factors, including severe fluid retention, advancing proliferative retinopathy despite laser therapy, and intrauterine growth retardation. Although the caesarean section rate in women with diabetes has fallen, the rate remains substantially higher than that of the background population. In women with diabetic nephropathy, the rate of caesarean section in most series was even higher. Kitzmiller *et al.*[50] reported 80%, Grenfell *et al.*[46] 73% and Dicker *et al.*[52] 75%. The average was approximately 75%, although, in the total diabetic population for most series, the caesarean section rate is around 45%. Only Drury[4] has reported a much lower caesarean section rate for diabetic women.

Part of the reason for the increased rate in diabetic pregnancy may be the timing of delivery to effect fetal rescue, since, in many reports, the mean gestation was around 35 weeks. In contrast, Jovanovic and Jovanovic[49] have reported a mean gestation of 40 weeks in 8 women with nephropathy who had been normoglycaemic prior to and throughout pregnancy. Estimation of amniotic fluid phosphatidyl glycerol provides some information about fetal lung maturity and it may be, in future, that amniotic fluid erythropoietin and C-peptide will give information on fetal hypoxia and fetal overstimulation, respectively, but there is no experience of such techniques in women with nephropathy. In recent years, with the advent of improved maternal glycaemic control, neonatal respiratory distress syndrome has become less frequent. During delivery, normal blood glucose levels are maintained by the continuous infusion of dextrose and insulin.

Insulin requirements drop dramatically to prepregnancy levels following delivery of the placenta.

INFANT OF A DIABETIC MOTHER (IDM)

At delivery, fetal metabolism and physiology should have been programmed to allow adequate extraction of oxygen from the environment and energy substrates from endogenous stores until feeding begins[1]. In the fetus and the newborn infant of the diabetic mother, the ability of the fetus to initiate these functions depends on the maturity of the fetal lungs at the time of delivery and the preceding intrauterine metabolic milieu which presets neonatal endogenous insulin secretion. Careful monitoring in a special neonatal unit with experienced neonatal paediatricians allows identification and appropriate management of respiratory or metabolic aberrations in such infants. Because of the occasional need to deliver diabetic women early, respiratory distress syndrome has been reported on average to affect about 20% of babies. During the 1970s and 80s, there has been a significant decrease in both the incidence of and mortality from respiratory problems due to improvements in maternal metabolic control, later delivery and improvements in neonatal care. If fetal hyperinsulinaemia has been stimulated by poor maternal metabolic control, fetal surfactant production may be impaired because of diminished incorporation of choline into lecithin; thus, respiratory distress may develop even at or beyond the 37th week of gestation. However, the neonate of the diabetic woman with nephropathy may be partially protected from the respiratory distress syndrome due to the earlier appearance of phospholipids, such as phosphidyl glycerol and saturated phosphatidyl choline, during such complicated pregnancies – possibly because of an adrenal cortical response induced by stress.

The metabolism of glucose, ketone bodies, lipids and amino acids in the infant undergoes major change just after delivery. In the offspring of a diabetic woman, a rapid fall of blood glucose within 30–60 min of delivery relates to neonatal hyperinsulinaemia. Pederson's elegant studies showed that mean blood glucose in the first day of life is inversely correlated with the maternal mean blood glucose level during the final months of pregnancy[54]. Pederson proposed a hypothesis that maternal hyperglycaemia stimulates fetal and immediate postnatal hyperinsulinaemia in the newborn IDM. This has been supported by histological studies showing β-cell hyperplasia and by direct measurement of plasma insulin levels in the newborn of women with IDM[53]. In the inadequately controlled pregnant diabetic woman, fetal hyperinsulinism may account for prolonged hypoglycaemia persisting for 24–48 h in the neonate. Prompt recognition and early treatment of symptomatic hypoglycaemia in the newborn should minimize sequelae. The Pederson hypothesis has been extended by Freinkel *et al.*[55] to include, not only glucose, but also amino acids, free fatty acids and glycerol which promote fetal hyperinsulinaemia and subsequent macrosomia.

The aetiology of macrosomia in diabetic pregnancy is probably multifactorial. The infant of the poorly regulated diabetic mother in class A-D will be macrosomic, as compared with the infant of the well-controlled diabetic or non-diabetic mother. This macrosomia indicates, not only an excess of subcutaneous tissue, but also hypertrophy and hyperplasia of visceral organs, such as heart and liver. Macrosomia may be related to the total amount of substrates crossing the placenta, rather than any one individual energy substrate; such substrate would include glucose, glycerol, amino acids and free fatty acids. Clinical consequences of macrosomia may be difficult vaginal deliveries due to shoulder girdle dystocia and birth asphyxia or injury which may cause long-term sequelae. The offspring of mothers with diabetic nephropathy, in contrast to infants of other diabetic mothers, tend to be light for gestational age, rather than macrosomic. Mean birthweight in Jovanovic and Jovanovic's study[49] was 3100 g, Grenfell *et al.*[46] 2800 g and Dicker *et al.*[52] 2900 g. In most reports, birthweight was related to renal function, i.e. creatinine clearance, and hypertension. However, in Jovanovic's study, a relationship was found between birthweight and glycaemic control. Other neonatal problems associated with IDM are polycythaemia and hyperbilirubinaemia which is thought to be related to fetal hypoxia. An elevated level of umbilical cord erythropoietin, which is stimulated by hypoxia, was found in almost a fifth of IDM compared with the range of normal newborns and infants[56]. Polycythaemia of IDM may account for some cardiorespiratory problems, such as transient cardiomegaly.

In conclusion, with present day management strategies, perinatal mortality in women with diabetic nephropathy remains low and 3 recent series from London[46] (number of patients = 22), New York[49] (number of patients = 8) and Israel[52] (number of patients = 4) reported zero perinatal mortality. Infants of such mothers had neonatal problems, including respiratory distress syndrome and congenital abnormalities, but such problems can be reduced by maintaining a normal blood glucose. There is good evidence to suggest that in future these may be avoidable by good metabolic control, particularly during embryogenesis but also continued throughout pregnancy.

LONG-TERM MATERNAL HEALTH

Unfortunately, women with diabetic nephropathy have a relatively poor prognosis[20]. The disabling 'microvascular' and neurological diabetic complications include loss of vision, endstage renal failure, lesions of the foot and, to a lesser degree, autonomic neuropathy and postural hypotension. Myocardial infarction, partly related to non-diabetic risk factors, but undoubtedly enhanced by diabetes (hyperglycaemia and probably hyperinsulinaemia) is a leading cause of death in the diabetic adult[35,57]. Most of our information on the natural history of renal disease in IDDM comes from studies of patients attending large clinics[35]. The Steno Memorial Hospital in Denmark has recently reported on 1475 male and female patients diagnosed before 1953 who were aged less than 31 years at diagnosis and were followed for at least 25 years[20]. A total of 41% developed proteinuria after a median of 16 years. The risk of early death was substantially greater in patients with proteinuria. Thus, after 40 years duration, only 10% of patients with proteinuria survived compared with over 70% survival in patients free of proteinuria. Uraemia was the principal cause of death. Diabetic subjects now comprise up to 20–25% of subjects on dialysis and transplantation programmes. Many such patients, however, have multisystem complications and coronary heart disease is a major risk to their health. Coronary heart disease has been reported to be very much more common in patients with proteinuria[35,58,60] and risk factors for coronary heart disease, such as high blood pressure and higher serum cholesterol levels, are found in this group. From a preventive point of view, it is important, therefore, that young mothers with diabetic nephropathy have optimal diabetic control, treatment for hyperlipidaemia, and control of hypertension[59]. They should be strongly encouraged to be non-smokers and of ideal body weight.

These measures, however, may not necessarily improve the excess mortality in this high-risk group. When, in 1986, Grenfell *et al.* studied the longer term outlook of 15 women documented as having diabetogenic proteinuria during pregnancy between 1974–1984, one patient had already died, one was awaiting renal transplantation and two had mild, yet significant, renal failure[46]. In the transplant patients reported by Ogburn *et al.*[36], one patient died during pregnancy, one woman died 12 years after pregnancy, spontaneous weight-bearing fractures occurred in two patients and visual impairment was present in five cases.

It is essential, therefore, that the longer term aspects of the health of these women should be kept in mind when giving prepregnancy advice and when discussing the advisability of continuing with a pregnancy. Management of the consequences of proliferative retinopathy and endstage renal failure are a major disruption to family and personal lifestyle. If a woman decides to proceed with pregnancy, with present management strategies, the chances of a successful outcome are considerably better than they were in the past. This depends on high motivation and intensive effort on the part of the woman in a partnership with her caring team of obstetrician, physician and paediatrician.

CONCLUSION

Women with diabetes mellitus and renal impairment are identified as a particularly high-risk group, but, with careful combined supervision prior to and during pregnancy, a successful outcome can often be achieved. Prepregnancy counselling is particularly important, firstly to consider the advisability of pregnancy and secondly to optimize metabolic control prior to conception.

Acknowledgements

The authors are deeply grateful to Mrs Sandra A. Anderson for assistance in the preparation of the manuscript.

REFERENCES

1. Sutherland, H.W. and Stowers, J.M. (1984). *Carbohydrate Metabolism in Pregnancy and the Newborn.* (Edinburgh: Churchill Livingstone)
2. Hadden, D. R. (1986). Diabetes in pregnancy 1985. *Diabetologia,* **29,** 1–9
3. Molsted-Pedersen, L. and Kuhl, C. (1986). Obstetrical management in pregnancy. The Copenhagen Experience. *Diabetologia,* **29,** 13–16
4. Drury, M.I. (1986). Management of the pregnant diabetic patients – are the pundits right? *Diabetologia,* **29,** 10–12
5. National Diabetes Data Group (1979). Classification and diagnosis of diabetes and other categories of glucose intolerance. *Diabetes,* **28,** 1039–1057
6. Gorsuch, A.M., Lister, J., Dean, B.M., Spencer, K.M., McNally, J.M., Bottazzo, J.F. and Cudworth, A.G. (1981). Evidence for a long pre diabetic period in type I (insulin dependent) diabetes mellitus. *Lancet,* **2,** 1363–1365
7. Johnston, C., Yook, D.A., Cudworth, A.G. and Wolfe, E. (1983). HLA DR typing in identical twins with insulin dependent diabetes: difference between concordant and discordant pairs. *Br. Med. J.,* **286,** 253–256
8. Yoon, J.W., Austin, M., Onidara, T. and Notkins, A.L. (1979). Virus induced diabetes mellitus; isolation of a virus from the pancreas of a child with diabetic ketoacidosis. *N. Engl. J. Med.,* **300,** 1173–1179
9. Helgason, T. and Jonasson, M.R. (1981). Evidence for a food additive as a cause of ketosis prone diabetes. *Lancet,* **2,** 716–720
10. Toliona, A., Onodera, T., Yoon, J.W. and Notkins, A.L. (1980). Induction of diabetes by cumulative environmental insults from viruses and chemicals. *Nature (London),* **288,** 383–385
11. Lernmark, A., Haggloff, B., Freedman, Z., Irvine, J., Ludvigsson, J. and Holmgren, G. (1981). A prospective analysis of antibodies reacting with pancreatic islet cells in insulin dependent diabetic children. *Diabetologia,* **20,** 4, 471–474
12. Sensi, M., Poxolli, P., Gorsuch, A.N., Bottazzo, G.F. and Cudworth, A.G. (1981). Increased killer cell activity in insulin dependent (type I) diabetes mellitus. *Diabetologia,* **20,** 106–109
13. De Fronzo, R. and Ferranini, E. (1982). The pathogenesis of non insulin dependent diabetes: an update. *Medicine (Baltimore),* **61,** 125–140
14. Keen, H. and Jarrett, J. (1982). *Complications of Diabetes,* 2nd Edn. (London: Edward Arnold)
15. Stewart-Brown, S., Haslem, M. and Butler, N. (1983). Evidence for increasing prevalence of diabetes mellitus in childhood. *Br. Med. J.,* **286,** 1855–1857
16. Rodmann, H.M. (1979). Diabetic nephropathy. Impact on the prognosis of the pregnant diabetic woman. In Merkatz, I.R. and Adam, P.A.J. (eds.) *The Diabetic Pregnancy. A Perinatal Perspective.* pp. 57–71. (New York: Grune and Stratton)

17. Furhrmann, K., Reiher, H., Semmler, K., Fischer, F., Fischer, M. and Glockner, E. (1983). Prevention of congenital malformations in infants of insulin dependent diabetic mothers. *Diabetes Care*, **6,** 219–223
18. Steel, J.M., Johnstone, F.D., Smith, A.F. and Duncan, L.J.P. (1984). Pre-preg nancy clinic approach. In Sutherland, H.W. and Stowers, J.M. (eds.) *Carbohydrate Metabolism in Pregnancy and the Newborn*, pp. 75–86. (Churchill Livingstone)
19. Hytten, F. and Chamberlain, G. (1980). *Clinical Physiology in Obstetrics*. (Oxford: Blackwell Scientific Publications)
20. Andersen, A.R., Christiansen, J.S., Andersen, J.K., Kreiner, S. and Deckert, T. (1983). Diabetic nephropathy in type I (insulin dependent) diabetes: an epidemiological study. *Diabetologia*, **25,** 496–501
21. Christiansen, J.S. (1985). Glomerular hyperfiltration in diabetes mellitus. *Diabetic Med.*, **2,** 235–239
22. Parving, H.H., Nower, I., Kehlet, H., Morgensen, C.E., Fendsen, P.A.A. and Heading, L.G. (1977). The effect of short term glucagon infusion on kidney function in normal man. *Diabetologia*, **13,** 323–325
23. Christiansen, J.S., Gammelgaarde, J., Franzsen, M., Orskoff, H. and Parving, H.H. (1982). Kidney function and size in type I diabetic patients before and during growth hormone administration for one week. *Diabetologia*, **22,** 333–337
24. Viberti, G. and Keen, H. (1984). The patterns of proteinuria in diabetes mellitus – relevance to pathogenesis and prevention of diabetic nephropathy. *Diabetes*, **33,** 686–692
25. Viberti, G., Pickup, J.C., Jarrett, R.J. and Keen, H. (1979). Effect of control of blood glucose on urinary excretion of albumin and beta 2 microglobulin in insulin dependent diabetes. *N. Engl. J. Med.*, **300,** 638–641
26. Viberti, G.C., Wiseman, M.J. and Bending, J.J. (1986). Prevention of diabetic nephropathy: markers of disease and perspectives for intervention. *Diabetic Med.*, **3,** 208–211
27. Bell, E.T. (1953). Renal vascular disease in diabetes mellitus. *Diabetes*, **2,** 376–389
28. Mauer, S.M., Barbosa, J. and Vernier, R.L. (1976). Development of diabetic vascular lesions in normal kidneys transplanted into patients with diabetes mellitus. *N. Engl. J. Med.*, **295,** 916–920
29. Bloodworth, J.M.B., Engerman, R.L. and Anderson, P.J. (1973). Microangiopathy in the experimentally diabetic animal. In Calmerini-Davalos, R.A. and Cole, H.S. (eds.) *Vascular and Neurological Changes in Early Diabetes*, pp. 245. (New York: Academic Press)
30. Bunn, F.H. (1981). Evaluation of glycosylated haemoglobin in diabetic patients. *Diabetes*, **30,** 613–617
31. Stevens, V.J., Rouzer, C.A., Monnier, V.M. and Cerami, A. (1978). Diabetic cataract formation: role of glycosylation of lens crystallins. *Proc. Natl. Acad. Sci.*, **75,** 2918–2922
32. Schnider, S.L. and Kohn, R.R. (1980). Glycosylation of human collagen in aging and diabetes mellitus. *J. Clin. Invest.*, **66,** 1179–1181
33. Kennedy, L., Mehl, T.D., Elder, E., Varghese, M. and Merinee, T.J. (1982). Nonenzymatic glycosylation of serum and plasma proteins. *Diabetes*, **31,** (Suppl. 3), 52–56
34. Witztum, J.L., Mahoney, E.M., Branks, M.J., Fisher, M., Elam, R. and Steinberg,

D. (1982). Non-enzymatic glycosylation of low density lipoprotein alters its biologic activity. *Diabetes*, **31,** 283–291
35. Jensen, T., Borch-Johnsten, K., Kofoed-Enevoldsen, A. and Deckert, T. (1987). Coronary heart disease in young type I (insulin dependent) diabetic patients with and without diabetic nephropathy: incidence and risk factors. *Diabetologia*, **30,** 144–148
36. Ogburn, P.L., Kitzmiller, J.L., Hare, J.W., Phillippe, M., Gabbe, S.G., Miodovnik, M., Tagatz, G.E., Nagal, T.G., Williams, P.P., Goetz, F.C., Barbosa, J.J. and Sutherland, D.F. (1986). Pregnancy following renal transplantation in Class T diabetes mellitus. *J. Am. Med. Assoc.*, **255,** 911–915
37. Reece, E.A., Egan, J.F.X., Coustan, D.R., Tamborlane, W., Bates, S.E., O'Neil, T. and Fitzpatrick, J.G. (1985). Coronary artery disease in diabetic pregnancy. *Am. J. Obstet. Gynaecol.*, **154/1,** 150–151
38. Pedersen, J.F., Molsted-Pedersen, L. and Mortensen, H.B. (1984). Fetal growth delay and maternal hemoglobin A1C in early diabetic pregnancy. *Obstet. Gynaecol.*, **64,** 351–356
39. Hare, J.W. and White, P. (1980). Gestational diabetes and White Classification. *Diabetes Care*, **3,** 2, 394
40. Lind, T. and Anderson, J. (1984). Does random blood glucose sampling outdate testing for glycosuria in the detection of diabetes during pregnancy? *Br. Med. J.*, **289,** 1569–1571
41. Freinkel, N. (1985). Proceedings of the Second International Workshop-Conference on gestational diabetes mellitus. *Diabetes*, **34,** (suppl. 2), 1–130
42. Mylvaganam, R., Stowers, J.M., Steel, J.M., Wallace, J., MacHendry, J.C. and Wright, A.D. (1983). Insulin immunogenicity in pregnancy: maternal and fetal studies. *Diabetologia*, **24,** 19–25
43. Serup, L. (1986). Influence of pregnancy on diabetic retinopathy. *Acta Endocrinol. Suppl.*, **277,** 122–124
44. Phelps, R.L., Sakol, P., Metzger, B.M., Jampol, L.M., Frienkel, N. (1986). Changes in diabetic nephropathy during pregnancy. *Arch. Ophthalmol.*, **104,** 1806–1810
45. Wright, A., Steel, P., Bennett, J.R., Watts, G. and Polak, A. (1987). The urinary excretion of albumin in normal pregnancy. *Br. J. Obstet. Gynaecol.*, **94,** 408–412
46. Grenfell, A., Brudenell, J.M., Doddridge, M.C. and Watkins, P.J. (1986). Pregnancy in diabetic women who have proteinuria. *Q. J. Med.*, **59,** 379–386
47. Nesler, C.L., Sinclair, S.H., Swartz, S.S. and Gabbe, S.J. (1985). Diabetic nephropathy in pregnancy. *Clin. Obstet. Gynaecol.*, **28,** 528
48. Diamond, M.P., Shah, D.M., Hester, R.A., Vaughn, W.K., Cotton, R.B. and Boehm, F.H. (1985). Complication of insulin dependent diabetic pregnancies by pre eclampsia and/or chronic hypertension: analysis of outcome. *Am. J. Perinatol.*, **2,** 263–267
49. Jovanovic, R. and Jovanovic, L. (1984). Obstetric management when normoglycaemia is maintained in diabetic pregnant women with vascular compromise. *Am. J. Obstet. Gynaecol.*, **149,** 617–623
50. Kitzmiller, J.L., Brown, E.R., Phillippe, M., Stark, A.R., Acker, D., Kaldany, A., Singh, S. and Hare, J.W. (1981). Diabetic nephropathy and perinatal outcome. *Am. J. Obstet. Gynaecol.*, **147,** 741–751
51. Hare, J.W. and White, P. (1977). Pregnancy in diabetes complicated by vascular disease. *Diabetes*, **26,** 953–955

52. Dicker, D., Feldberg, D., Peleg, D., Karp, M. and Goldman, J.A. (1986). Pregnancy complicated by diabetic nephropathy. *J. Perinatol. Med.*, **14,** 299–305
53. Persson, B., Heding, L.G., Lunell, N.O., Psechera, H., Stangenberg, M. and Wagner, J. (1982). Fetal beta cell function in diabetic pregnancy. *Am. J. Obstet. Gynaecol.*, **144,** 455–459
54. Pedersen, J. (1975). Fetal macrosomia. In Sutherland, H.W. and Stowers, J.M. (eds.) *Carbohydrate Metabolism in Pregnancy and the Newborn.* pp. 127–139. (Edinburgh: Churchill Livingstone)
55. Freinkel, N., Phelps, R.E. and Betzger, B.E. (1978). Intermediary metabolism during normal pregnancy. In Sutherland, H.W. and Stowers, J.M. (eds.) *Carbohydrate Metabolism in Pregnancy and the Newborn.* pp. 1–31. (Basle: Springer Verlag)
56. Widness, J.A., Susa, J.B., Garcia, J.F., Singer, D.B., Sengal, P., Ol, W., Schwartz, R. and Schwartz, H.C. (1981). Increased erythropoietin in infants born to diabetic mothers and in hyperinsulinaemic rhesus fetuses. *J. Clin. Invest.*, **67,** 637–642
57. Turnbridge, W.M.G. (1981). Factors contributing to deaths of diabetics under 50 years of age. *Lancet*, **2,** 569–572
58. Borch-Johnsen, K. and Kreiner, S. (1987). Proteinuria – value as a predictor of cardiovascular mortality in insulin dependent diabetes mellitus. *Br. Med. J.*, **294,** 1651–1654
59. Parving, H.H., Andersen, A.R., Smidt, U.M., Hommel, E., Mathiesen, E.R. and Svendsen, P.A. (1987). The effect of antihypertensive treatment on kidney function in diabetic nephropathy. *Br. Med. J.*, **294,** 1443–1447
60. Jensen, T., Borch-Johnsen, K., Kofoed-Enevoldsen, A. and Deckert, T. (1987). Coronary heart disease in young type I (insulin dependent) diabetic patients with and without diabetic nephropathy: incidence and risk factors. *Diabetologia*, **30,** 144–148

5

COLLAGEN VASCULAR DISEASES

A. M. MACLEOD

Collagen vascular diseases are a group of relatively unusual conditions which involve many organs, including the kidney. The commonest is systemic lupus erythematosus (SLE), and others which affect the kidney include polyarteritis nodosa and scleroderma (progressive systemic sclerosis). Pregnancy was formerly ill-advised in all these conditions but over the last decade it has been successful in women with SLE and is now discouraged only in specific circumstances. In the other less common multisystem diseases, however, the prognoses for both mother and baby remain poor.

SYSTEMIC LUPUS ERYTHEMATOSUS

In SLE, autoantibodies form immune complexes with nuclear antigens – principally DNA. These complexes are deposited in blood vessel walls, including those in the glomerulus, complement is activated and tissue is damaged by the subsequent inflammatory process.

Pathology

Most of the histological patterns seen in the primary glomerulonephritides can be found in SLE but certain characteristic forms do occur (Table 5.1). Generally, the degree of clinical renal impairment is reflected in the severity of the histological changes at the time of biopsy. The pathological abnormalities may change, however, and, in some cases, a progressive deterioration occurs.

Ginzler *et al.*[1] reported that nine of 31 patients originally showing focal proliferative glomerular lesions developed a progressive form of diffuse glomerular disease between one and twelve years after the initial biopsy diagnosis. A further group[2], who described 31 of their own patients as well as reviewing three other series, noted that the prognostic information from renal biopsies was of less value than the simplest clinical estimations of renal function. More recently, a study of 102 patients[3] confirmed that clinical factors were paramount in predicting the outcome of lupus nephropathy. Men, those whose serum creatinine was elevated, and patients in whom the diagnosis was made before the age of 24 have a particularly poor prognosis. The investigators did find, however, that the presence of glomerulosclerosis, fibrous crescents, interstitial fibrosis and tubular atrophy were also indicative of disease progression. One study of women who had been previously pregnant indicated that biopsies taken immediately postpartum showed more severe histological lesions than had been detected on earlier occasions[4].

Early clinical studies

The majority of early reports described pregnancy in patients with SLE affecting any organ – not specifically the kidney[5–14]; the number

TABLE 5.1 Types of glomerulonephritis observed in patients with systemic lupus erythematosus

Minimal change glomerulonephritis
Mild mesangial proliferative glomerulonephritis
Focal proliferative glomerulonephritis
Membranous glomerulonephritis
Diffuse proliferative glomerulonephritis
– including crescent formation

of patients with documented nephropathy in each study was therefore small. As tests of kidney function were less accurate and biopsy less frequently performed than in recent years, renal involvement was generally recognized only when relatively severe. Furthermore, few studies described treatment regimes, in particular the use of corticosteroids. Most authors noted that pregnancy was most hazardous in their patients with SLE when the kidney was affected and they concluded that pregnancy was contraindicated in such women. One report[5] emphasized progression of the disease postpartum in patients with renal lupus although no data on renal function prior to pregnancy were given. Estes and Larson[6] described 10 pregnancies in nine women with lupus nephritis. Half these pregnancies ended in fetal death, and, in all cases, the renal disease progressed during pregnancy. Two women died in renal failure within one year of delivery, but, in the other seven, renal function remained stable or improved postpartum. Coexisting hypertension indicated the poorest prognosis for both pregnancy and renal function. Garsenstein *et al.*[7] followed 33 women with SLE during pregnancy and noted that all four who died despite steroid therapy had histological evidence of renal involvement. In that study also, however, three live full-term babies were born to women with lupus nephritis despite severe changes on renal biopsy; the authors do point out that these three women had serum urea nitrogen concentrations of less than 30 mg/100 ml (10 mmol/L).

Deterioration of renal function during pregnancy was noted in over half the patients with renal SLE in one study[8], but, in only two of 12, in another[9]. A high incidence of maternal death was reported by some[6,7] but this was not confirmed by others[10,11]. Some years later, it was noted[12] that there was no significant difference in death rates between pregnant and non-pregnant patients with lupus nephropathy.

Since pregnancy appeared hazardous, therapeutic abortion was frequently advocated in women with lupus nephritis. In one study[13], four of 12 women died following the procedure and others reported a decrease in renal function[5,7–9]. Thus, termination of pregnancy did not appear to have a beneficial effect on lupus nephritis, although a more recent study[14] indicated that such surgery can be tolerated if large doses of corticosteroids are given.

These early reports were inconclusive and, in some areas, contradictory. By the end of the 1970s, the need for more detailed studies of larger numbers of patients with SLE involving the kidneys was clear. In particular, the effect of the disease on the pregnancy and fetal outcome as well as the influence of pregnancy on the course of the disease required evaluation so that patients could be advised and managed more appropriately.

Clinical studies performed from 1980

From 1980 onwards, several groups studied women with renal lupus during and after pregnancy. Some of these were multicentre studies which allowed firmer conclusions to be drawn from observing larger numbers of patients. The two main issues addressed were the influence of SLE with renal involvement on both the pregnancy and the fetus and the effect of pregnancy on the subsequent course of lupus nephropathy.

Outcome of pregnancy in women with lupus nephropathy

The first major comprehensive study[15] followed 65 pregnancies in 47 women. In 35 women, the diagnosis of lupus nephropathy was made on renal biopsy; the remaining 12 who also had established SLE showed haematuria, proteinuria or abnormal renal function. In 31 pregnancies where there was no clinical evidence of active SLE (either renal or systemic) for the six months prior to pregnancy and the serum creatinine concentration during this time was normal, the rate of live births was 88% and the number of premature births the same as in the normal population. There were three spontaneous abortions, two during the second trimester, and, since this was greater than expected, the overall success rate was reduced by 8%. These results are similar to those of normotensive pregnant women who have other types of renal parenchymal disease with normal renal function[16,17]. An exacerbation of SLE occurred during pregnancy or postpartum in 10 of the 31 cases studied. This was reflected in a higher incidence of hypertension and proteinuria in late pregnancy but all the pregnancies, other than one which was electively terminated, ended successfully.

The live birth rate in the 23 pregnancies where SLE was clinically active in the six months before pregnancy was 64%; 24% less than the group without active disease during that time. One pregnancy loss, a spontaneous abortion at seven weeks, was thought to be within the expected rate but the other seven were judged to be due to disease activity. Only two of these women had an abnormal serum creatinine concentration prior to pregnancy, but, in five, the creatinine became abnormal during pregnancy and there was one maternal death. Of nine further patients in whom the diagnosis of SLE was made during pregnancy, there were five live births, one stillbirth, two spontaneous abortions and one elective termination of pregnancy; one mother died of pancreatitis 18 months after delivery.

Overall, this study indicates that women with SLE whose disease is inactive for six months prior to conception are very likely to have a successful pregnancy with a normal full-term baby. The chances of a favourable outcome are less if the disease is active immediately before pregnancy or the diagnosis is made during pregnancy.

Similar results were reported in the same year by Houser and colleagues[18] in 18 pregnancies in 11 women with known lupus nephritis, 10 of whom had a biopsy proven diagnosis. Of those whose GFR was over 90 ml/min, all 12 delivered live children; 11 at term and one at 36 weeks by caesarian section. Six patients had a GFR of less than 90 ml/min. Two delivered live infants, three suffered spontaneous abortion and one underwent elective termination in the tenth week of pregnancy.

A further study[19] from California gave fewer details of the pregnancies and neonatal outcome and did not comment on the basis for the diagnosis of lupus nephropathy. The authors reported that 28 of 38 (74%) women in whom the creatinine clearance was over 80 ml/min prior to pregnancy, delivered live infants, whereas only 9 of 14 (64%) of those with clearances between 50–80 ml/min had pregnancies which ended successfully. The success rate, therefore, again reflected renal function before pregnancy.

A French group[20] investigated a slightly different group of 36 women, 31 of whom had biopsy-proven nephritis. In 69 of the 104 gestations, the diagnosis of SLE was made at least three months after delivery. If four women who underwent therapeutic abortion are excluded, 83% of these patients who were diagnosed postpartum had successful pregnancies. As noted by others[13], all those pregnancies in which SLE was in remission prior to conception ended successfully whereas only 66% of women with active disease before pregnancy and 60% of those in whom the diagnosis was made during pregnancy gave birth to live infants. No comment was made in this study about any obstetric complications.

In 1984, Imbasciati and colleagues[4] reported 26 pregnancies in 19 women, all of whom had biopsy-proven lupus nephritis. If three women who underwent therapeutic abortion are excluded, 62.5% of pregnancies were successful, indicating that the overall outcome is less favourable in this study than in others[15,18–20]. In eight of the 26 cases, the diagnosis of SLE was made during pregnancy but the number of successful pregnancies in this subgroup is not stated. Other investigators[14] have shown that such women are less likely to deliver live infants than those in whom the diagnosis is made prior to conception. The reason for this is unclear but it may be that it takes some time for an appropriate treatment regime to be established and bring the recently diagnosed lupus under control. All but two of the patients had an exacerbation of SLE during pregnancy; a higher incidence than that found by others[15,18–20]. The authors themselves suggest that the low doses of corticosteroids given to treat these exacerbations were probably inadequate. Taken together, these factors may explain why the outcome of pregnancy was less successful in the patients reported in this study.

Overall, therefore, women with lupus nephritis without evidence of active disease before conception, although less likely to have a successful pregnancy than the normal population, do have a 70–80% chance of delivering a live child. If SLE is active prior to pregnancy or develops during pregnancy, this chance is considerably diminished.

The effects of pregnancy on the course of lupus nephropathy

The larger more recent studies[14,15,18–20] monitored the effect of pregnancy on activity of the renal and extrarenal manifestations of SLE. One group[15] showed that 68% of those whose disease was in remission prior to conception remained in remission during pregnancy and the postpartum period. There was an exacerbation of lupus nephropathy in 10 patients (32%) and five of those also showed evidence of systemic activity. Half the patients had not had renal function measured in the six months prior to conception and three of the five had serum creatinine levels over 300 μmol/L during pregnancy. Blood pressure recordings were noted for seven patients and all were hypertensive during pregnancy with diastolic blood pressure in excess of 100 mmHg. Other evidence of renal involvement included increased proteinuria and haematuria; two patients developed nephrotic syndrome. Eight of the 10 patients were treated with corticosteroids, chloroquine or cyclophosphamide although the dosage regimens were not stated and the eight patients followed for three months or more underwent complete or partial reversal of the exacerbation of their disease.

SLE was active in 25 patients prior to conception. In 10, the clinical manifestations remained unchanged, in three, they improved, but, in 12, they worsened. Of these 12, five showed a decline in renal function and one died; six had evidence of disease in other organs. Eleven were treated with corticosteroids with or without cytotoxic agents, and, in eight followed for over two months, there was a reversal of both renal and extrarenal manifestations of disease activity.

These data require cautious interpretation for two reasons. Firstly, the incidence of exacerbation as a result of pregnancy may have been exaggerated as the increased activity of SLE in some patients may merely have reflected the natural course of their disease. A rise in urinary protein excretion was classified as an increase in disease activity. A transient rise in proteinuria, however, without any alteration in the progression of disease has been recorded during pregnancy in women with primary renal disease[17]. Overall, therefore, the actual rate of exacerbation of SLE may have been overestimated.

The onset of SLE during pregnancy or the postpartum period was accompanied by significant maternal morbidity. Four of the nine patients developed nephrotic syndrome and three showed a marked decline in renal function; seven had manifestations of lupus affecting other organs. Five patients received steroids and seven underwent clinical remission. Whether pregnancy precipitated the onset of SLE was unclear but the subsequent course of the disease was probably no different from that expected in the absence of pregnancy; moreover, five of the nine patients subsequently experienced uncomplicated pregnancies.

Another study[18], although smaller, largely confirmed that of Hayslett and Lynn[15]. Eighteen pregnancies were reported in 11 women with lupus nephritis. Five women, four of whom had active disease at the onset of pregnancy, suffered an exacerbation of their renal disease during pregnancy. Three of the five patients showed a deterioration in renal function and all showed hypertension and increased proteinuria. All of the patients, with one exception, were treated with prednisolone or cytotoxic drugs during pregnancy and high-dose oral prednisolone at the time of delivery. The renal disease did not follow a rapidly progressive course and, in a follow-up period which varied from four months to 12 years, none of the patients died or required treatment for endstage renal disease.

Others[20] confirmed the clear influence of the clinical activity of SLE before conception. Exacerbation was observed in 11 of 15 pregnancies occurring in patients with acute SLE although worsening of renal disease was noted in only three; one patient developed nephrotic syndrome and acute renal failure which did not recover and she required long-term haemodialysis. SLE was diagnosed during pregnancy or in the postpartum period in nine patients. Three developed nephrotic syndrome and two had abnormal renal function. Seven were treated with prednisone and, at follow up, were noted to be in remission; the two untreated patients suffered frequent relapses. Eleven women became pregnant after at least five months of complete clinical remission of active disease and only one suffered an exacerbation of lupus nephropathy. Similar results have been reported by others[15,18].

Fine and colleagues[19] monitored renal function for between three and 12 months postpartum in 52 pregnancies. In 38, creatinine clearance prior to pregnancy was normal or minimally impaired (i.e. >80 ml/min). Thirty patients (79%) showed no change in renal function postpartum, five (13%) suffered a transient and three (8%) a persistent decline in renal function. When prepregnancy creatinine clearance was between 50–80 ml/min, 10 of 14 (71%) patients had stable renal function at follow up, two (14%) showed a transient and two (14%) a persistent decline in renal function. Renal function after pregnancy thus reflected that prior to conception.

A further study, published in 1984[4], which showed a lower incidence of successful pregnancy in women with lupus nephropathy also showed that, in 17 of the 19 mothers, renal function declined during pregnancy. Four developed acute renal failure and two died. In this study, however, all but two patients had active lupus nephropathy during pregnancy and these exacerbations may have been treated by inadequate doses of corticosteroids.

In summary, deterioration of renal function during and after pregnancy is influenced primarily by the degree of renal impairment and disease activity before conception. In addition there is some evidence that aggressive treatment of exacerbations of SLE during pregnancy with corticosteroids may prevent subsequent worsening of lupus nephropathy.

Renal histology and clinical outcome in lupus nephropathy

One study[21] set out with the particular objective of relating the outcome of pregnancy to the abnormalities noted on renal biopsy in patients with lupus nephropathy. Fifteen patients who had 20 pregnancies after the onset of SLE were studied. Biopsies were taken between three months and eight years prior to pregnancy with 12 of the 15 being performed within the two years prior to conception. There was no correlation between the severity of histological change and either the outcome of pregnancy or subsequent deterioration in renal function. The majority of those with diffuse proliferative or membranous changes had successful normal deliveries while spontaneous abortions and neonatal deaths were recorded in patients with minimal change or mesangial proliferative lesions. These investigators noted, as had others[15,18–20], that renal function before conception was a more accurate guide to both the future course of lupus nephropathy and the likelihood of a successful pregnancy.

There are two difficulties associated with relating biopsy changes to clinical outcome in pregnant women with renal lupus. Firstly, since the severity of lupus nephropathy may change spontaneously, biopsy appearances several months or years before pregnancy are unlikely to be representative of those immediately prior to conception. Secondly, histological features may be altered by drug therapy. One group[15] treated all patients who had diffuse proliferative features and subendothelial deposits noted on electron microscopy with corticosteroids, and subsequent biopsy invariably revealed a more benign lesion; this finding has been confirmed by other investigators[22].

It is difficult, therefore, to obtain information on the histological severity of lupus nephropathy immediately prior to pregnancy. In the absence of such data, renal function before conception appears to be a better indicator of prognosis for both pregnancy and renal disease in women with SLE than does previously noted histological change.

Management of lupus nephropathy in association with pregnancy

There are three main aims in managing pregnancy complicated by lupus nephropathy:

(1) To assess the activity of SLE and the severity of any renal impairment;
(2) To counsel the patient considering pregnancy;
(3) To treat lupus nephropathy during pregnancy and provide optimum obstetric care to patients with impaired renal function.

Assessment of activity of SLE and of renal function

The most frequently observed non-renal clinical features of active SLE are anaemia, thrombocytopenia, arthritis and vesicular or papular skin eruptions. Involvement of the kidneys in an exacerbation is suggested by a change in the urinary findings, particularly the onset of haematuria or a decline in renal function; an increase in proteinuria is a less reliable indication. Renal function should be assessed by regular monitoring of serum urea and creatinine concentrations or creatinine clearance.

Estimations of antibodies associated with SLE have been used to define disease activity. Neither the presence of antinuclear factors nor anti-DNA binding antibody, however, were found to be useful indicators of the outcome of pregnancy[23]: indeed, antinuclear factors have been detected in sera from between 1% and 5% of normal pregnant women[24,25]. Hypocomplementaemia, however, correlates well with increased activity of SLE during pregnancy[26]. The level of serum complement rises by 10% during pregnancy in patients with stable SLE compared with a rise of 25% in normal pregnant women[27].

These data were confirmed by others[28] who also showed, in a larger study, that women with known SLE who failed to show a rise in C3 or had declining levels during pregnancy suffered an increase in disease activity, obstetric complications and fetal morbidity and mortality. Furthermore, Devoe and Taylor[11] indicated that falling C3 levels correlated both with an exacerbation of SLE and with an increased rate of spontaneous abortion.

The presence of another serum factor, lupus anticoagulant, correlated with a high incidence of intrauterine fetal death in mid and late pregnancy[29,30]. A more recent study[31] evaluated the role of several serum factors during pregnancy complicated by SLE. Thrombocytopenia, proteinuria, hypocomplementaemia and the presence of circulating lupus anticoagulant were associated with increased fetal risk whereas titres of anti-DNA activity were of no value in predicting maternal or fetal outcome.

Counselling of patients with lupus nephropathy

Since most young women with SLE affecting the kidneys are regularly reviewed by renal physicians, pregnancy is often first discussed at a nephrology clinic. The patient can be advised that the majority of pregnancies in women with lupus nephropathy are successful and, if the disease is in remission for six months prior to conception and serum creatinine remains below 150 μmol/L, there is a 70–80% chance that a live child will be delivered. This applies even when marked renal and extrarenal manifestations were present at diagnosis and renal biopsy showed severe changes. The presence, however, of continued disease activity, worsening renal function or hypertension reduces the likelihood of an uncomplicated pregnancy. Continued care by an obstetrician, rheumatologist and nephrologist is helpful and fetal monitoring in the later stages of pregnancy may decrease the stillbirth rate. In addition, delivery should take place in a hospital with full neonatal intensive care facilities.

Treatment of lupus nephropathy during pregnancy

Corticosteroids and immunosuppressive drugs are the principal forms of treatment for lupus nephropathy. There is concern about the use of corticosteroids as toxic effects may occur at the dosages which are required to control the disease and some authors doubt their efficacy in treating the renal lesion[32] in the non-pregnant population. Immunosuppressive drugs have been shown to improve the prognosis in lupus nephropathy[33,34] although this has not been universally confirmed[35].

There is some reluctance to use corticosteroids and immunosuppressive drugs during pregnancy for fear of possible fetotoxic effects. Early animal studies showed an increased incidence of cleft palate in mice and rabbits[36,37]. A study[38] of 260 human pregnancies in which corticosteroids were given revealed no increase in congenital abnormalities and this was confirmed recently[39] in a survey of 490 pregnancies in women with renal transplants treated with prednisolone, azathioprine, cyclosporin A or combinations of these drugs. Rarely, masculinization of the female fetus has occurred[40] and, very occasionally, neonatal death from adrenocortical failure has been reported[41]. In addition, there is evidence that steroids do not cause fetal growth retardation[26,42]: children followed for between six months and eight years were of normal height and weight.

If SLE is in remission without treatment, corticosteroid therapy is not required during pregnancy. Early evidence[13] suggested that, if steroids were being given during pregnancy, a lower dose could control disease activity during the second trimester and therapy was unlikely to be required at all in the third trimester; an increased dosage, however, was necessary immediately postpartum. In a more recent study[43] of women with lupus nephropathy, steroid dosage was increased until serum complement levels returned to normal; if hypocomplementaemia persisted or renal function deteriorated, the dose was increased further. Intravenous steroids were given during labour and delivery. Using this regimen, fetal survival was 80% compared with 11% for those who had active disease during pregnancy and were not treated. Such increased corticosteroid dosages have been shown not to harm the fetus[26,44]. It appears, therefore, that corticosteroids are effective in treating active SLE involving the kidneys during pregnancy.

Immunosuppressive drugs, including azathioprine, cyclophosphamide and chlorambucil, have also been used to treat lupus nephropathy. One study[32] showed that renal biopsy changes improved to a greater extent when immunosuppressive drugs rather than corticosteroids were given. No comment, however, was made on renal function in these patients.

Azathioprine does cross the placenta but has been used successfully in pregnant patients with lupus nephropathy[18,19,45] and in pregnant renal transplant recipients[39] without an increase in fetal abnormality. Normal live births have been reported in women taking cyclophosphamide[18,45] and chlorambucil but these drugs are associated with the development of congenital abnormalities[46,47]. Plasmapheresis has been infrequently attempted in pregnant women with lupus nephropathy, and, while one group[48] found it improved vasculitis and decreased steroid requirements, another failed to confirm this[49].

In addition to drug therapy, patients with lupus nephropathy require close monitoring of blood pressure and renal function during pregnancy. Mild or moderate hypertension developing during pregnancy may be controlled by bed rest alone. One group[50] suggests that good initial control in severe hypertension can be obtained by parenteral hydralazine; methyldopa, however, remains the only antihypertensive whose long-term safety in pregnancy has been evaluated[51,52]. Oral hydralazine used alone can cause tachycardia, headaches and flushing and there is some evidence that uteroplacental perfusion is reduced[53]. While antihypertensive drugs are useful in prolonging pregnancy to allow fetal maturation, hypertension during late pregnancy which fails to respond to drug therapy is an indication for immediate delivery.

Renal function should be followed using serial serum creatinine or creatinine clearance estimations and the fetus monitored during the third trimester. Deterioration of renal function is an indication for hospital admission and the time of delivery judged according to the degree of hypertension, the rate of rise in serum creatinine concentration and the results of fetal monitoring. Haemodialysis has been used to treat a patient with severe renal impairment due to lupus nephropathy during pregnancy[54] with a successful outcome for herself and her baby. Renal transplantation has also been performed for endstage lupus nephropathy with subsequent successful pregnancy[55].

POLYARTERITIS NODOSA (PAN)

This rare condition affects at least twice as many men as women and has its onset most frequently during the sixth decade. Pregnancy is thus extremely unusual in patients with PAN. Renal involvement occurs in 60–90% of cases and can present with haematuria, proteinuria, hypertension or diminished renal function.

There are few studies of PAN during pregnancy. Mor-Joseph and colleagues reviewed nine case reports[56] and noted that both mothers in whom the diagnosis was made prior to pregnancy and who were treated with corticosteroids survived, as did their infants who were born at 34 and 37 weeks gestation. One patient died during the abortion of a 20-week fetus and another died six weeks after therapeutic termination of pregnancy. In the other six women, the diagnosis of PAN was made at autopsy up to six weeks postpartum; all the infants in this group survived. A further three women with quiescent disease and minimal renal involvement have had successful pregnancies[57].

There is insufficient evidence from the literature to comment on the advisability of pregnancy in women with stable treated PAN. Most authorities[56,57] suggest counselling women against pregnancy or suggesting therapeutic termination which appears to have less risk than a continuing pregnancy for the mother[58].

SCLERODERMA (Progressive Systemic Sclerosis)

This disorder of connective tissue involves principally the skin, lungs, heart, gastrointestinal tract and kidneys. It occurs mainly between the ages of 30 and 50; women are affected twice as often as men. The increased fibrosis in various organs is thought to be due to the overproduction of collagen but the aetiology and pathogenesis are unknown.

The combination of pregnancy and scleroderma is rare, both

because of the age of onset of the condition and because the patients tend to be relatively infertile[59,60]. A review of 21 case reports and two series[56] shows that, when scleroderma is diagnosed during pregnancy, the disease progresses rapidly. If there is renal or cardiac involvement, the risk of maternal death is high although most maternal deaths in women with scleroderma result from pulmonary complications or infection. An increased rate of spontaneous abortion is reported and the incidence of premature labour, stillbirth and perinatal mortality is high[59,61]. Since there is no known treatment for this condition and since maternal and fetal morbidity are high, pregnancy is not advised in women with scleroderma.

SUMMARY

(1) Patients with SLE in remission are likely to be fertile.

(2) Initial small studies of pregnancy in patients with SLE indicated the poorest prognosis for those with renal involvement.

(3) Large recent studies suggested that, if the disease was inactive and renal function normal before conception, the live birth rate was 70–80%; where SLE was active or renal function abnormal, the rate fell to around 60%.

(4) Renal function remains unchanged in approximately 60% pregnancies. Those in whom it deteriorates have generally had abnormal renal function often with hypertension prior to pregnancy.

(5) Therapeutic termination of pregnancy has no beneficial effect in lupus nephritis and is not advocated.

(6) Renal function is a better indicator of prognosis for both pregnancy and renal disease than the histological findings on renal biopsy.

(7) Hypocomplementaemia and the presence of lupus anticoagulant are indicators of high fetal morbidity and mortality.

(8) Treatment with corticosteroids is effective in active lupus

nephropathy during pregnancy and improves the prognosis for the fetus. There is no significant risk of fetotoxicity.

(9) Immunosuppressive drugs are effective during pregnancy but the administration of cyclophosphamide and chlorambucil is associated with the development of congenital abnormalities whereas azathioprine is not.

(10) Combined care of an obstetrician and nephrologist is advised for women with renal lupus during pregnancy. Hypertension requires control and renal function and fetal well-being, frequent monitoring. Delivery should take place in hospital with full neonatal facilities.

(11) Pregnancy in women with PAN is generally discouraged although some evidence suggests that pregnancy may be successful if the disease is stable and under treatment.

(12) The progression of scleroderma is hastened by pregnancy and both fetal and maternal morbidity are high. Pregnancy is therefore not advised.

REFERENCES

1. Ginzler, E.M., Nicastri, A.D., Chen, C-K., Freitlman, E.A., Diamond, H. and Kaplan, D. (1974). Progression of mesangial and focal to diffuse lupus nephritis. *N. Engl. J. Med.*, **279,** 693–696
2. Fries, J.F., Porta, J. and Liang, M.H. (1978). Marginal benefit of renal biopsy in systemic lupus erythematosus. *Arch. Int. Med.*, **138,** 1386–1389.
3. Austin, H.A., Muena, L.R., Joyce K.M., Antonovych, T.A., Kullick, M.E., Klippel, J.H., Decker, J.L. and Balour, J.E. (1983). Prognostic factors in lupus nephritis. *Am. J. Med.*, **75,** 382–391
4. Imbasciati, E., Surian, M., Bottino, S., Cosci, P., Colussi, G., Ambroso, G.C., Massa, I., Minetti, L., Pardi, G. and Ponticelli, C. (1984). Lupus nephropathy and pregnancy. *Nephron*, **36,** 46–51
5. Friedman, E.A. and Rutherford, J.W. (1956). Pregnancy and lupus erythematosus. *Obstet. Gynecol.*, **8,** 601–610
6. Estes, D. and Larson, D.L. (1965). Systemic lupus erythematosus and pregnancy. *Clin. Obstet. Gynecol.*, **8,** 307–321
7. Garsenstein, M., Pollak, V.E. and Kark, R.M. (1962). Systemic lupus erythematosus and pregnancy. *N. Engl. J. Med.*, **267,** 165–169
8. Boelaert, J., Morel-Maroger, L. and Mery, J-P. (1974). Renal insufficiency in lupus nephritis. *Adv. Nephrol.*, **4,** 249–252
9. Fairley, K.F., Whitworth, J.A. and Kincaid-Smith, P. (1973). Glomerulonephritis

in pregnancy. In Kincaid-Smith, P., Matthew, T.H. and Becker, E.L. (eds.) *Glomerulonephritis Morphology; Natural History and Treatment*, Part II, pp. 997–1025. (New York: John Wiley and Sons)

10. Dziubinski, E.H., Winkelmann, R.K. and Wilson, R.B. (1962). Systemic lupus erythematosus and pregnancy. *Am. J. Obstet. Gynecol.*, **84,** 1873–1877
11. Devoe, L.D. and Taylor, R.L. (1979). Systemic lupus erythematosus in pregnancy. *Am. J. Obstet. Gynecol.*, **135,** 473–479
12. Pollack, V.E., Pirani, C.L. and Schwartz, F.D. (1964). The natural history of the renal manifestations of systemic lupus erythematosus. *J. Lab. Clin. Med.*, **63,** 537–550
13. Donaldson, L.B. and de Alvarez, R. (1962). Further observations on lupus erythematosus associated with pregnancy. *Am. J. Obstet. Gynecol.*, **83,** 1461–1473
14. Bear, R.A. (1976). Pregnancy in patients with renal disease: a study of 44 cases. *Obstet. Gynecol.*, **48,** 13–18
15. Hayslett, J.P. and Lynn, R.I. (1980). Effect of pregnancy in patients with lupus nephropathy. *Kidney Int.*, **18,** 207–220
16. Ferris, T.F. (1975). Renal disease. In Burrow, G.N. and Ferris, T.S. (eds.) *Medical Complications During Pregnancy*, pp. 1–52. (Philadelphia: W.B. Saunders)
17. Strauch, B.S. and Hayslett, J.P. (1974). Kidney disease and pregnancy. *Br. Med. J.*, **4,** 578–582
18. Houser, M.T., Fish, A.J., Tagatz, G.E., Williams, P.P. and Michael, A.F. (1980). Pregnancy and systemic lupus erythematosus. *Am. J. Obstet. Gynecol.*, **138,** 409–413
19. Fine, L.G., Barnett, E.V., Danovitch, G.M., Nissenson, A.R., Connolly, M.E., Lieb, S.M. and Barrett, C.T. (1981). Systemic lupus erythematosus in pregnancy. *Ann. Intern. Med.*, **94,** 667–677
20. Jungers, P., Dougados, M., Pelissier, C., Kuttenn, F., Tron, F., Lesavre, P. and Bach, J-F. (1982). Lupus nephropathy and pregnancy. *Arch. Int. Med.*, **142,** 771–784
21. Devoe, L., Loy, G.L. and Spargo, B.H. (1983). Renal histology and pregnancy performance in systemic lupus erythematosus. *Clin. Exp. Hypertens.*, **B2,** 325–340
22. Hecht, B., Spiegel, N., Adler, M., Kashgarian, M. and Lett, J.P. (1976). Prognostic indices in lupus nephritis. *Medicine*, **55,** 163–181
23. Lubbe, W.F., Butler, W.S., Palmer, S.J. and Liggins, G.C. (1984). Lupus anticoagulant in pregnancy. *Br. J. Obstet. Gynaecol.*, **91,** 357–363
24. Reyes-Lopez, P.A., Santos, G. and Forsbach, G.B. (1980). Absence of ANA in pregnancy. *Arthrit. Rheum.*, **23,** 378
25. Hinkle, S.C., Merkatz, I.R., Gyves, M.T., Michel, B. and Moskowitz, R.W. (1979). Antinuclear factor and anti-DNA in sera of pregnant women. *Arthrit. Rheum.*, **22,** 201–202
26. Zurier, R.B., Argyros, T.G., Urman, J.D., Warren, J. and Rothfield, N.F. (1977). Systemic lupus erythematosus: Management during pregnancy. *Obstet. Gynecol.*, **51,** 178–180
27. Chetlin, S.M., Medsger, T.A., Cantas, S.N. and di Bartolones, A.G. (1977). Serum complement values during pregnancy in patients with systemic lupus erythematosus. *Arthrit. Rheum.*, **20,** 111
28. Ziegler, G. and Medsger, T.A. (1984). Serial complement levels of SLE pregnancies. *Arthrit. Rheum.*, **27,** 5130 (Apr. Suppl.)

29. Abramowsky, C.R., Vegas, M.E. and Swinehart, B.A. (1980). Decidual vasculopathy of the placenta in lupus erythematosus. *N. Engl. J. Med.*, **303,** 66–72
30. Boey, M.L., Colaco, C.B., Gharavi, A.E., Elkan, K.B., Loizou, S. and Hughes, G.R. (1983). Thrombosis in systemic lupus erythematosus: striking association with presence of circulating lupus anticoagulant. *Br. Med. J.*, **287,** 1021–1023
31. Lockshin, M.D., Harpal, P.C., Druzin, M.L., Becker, C.G., Klein, R.F., Watson, R.M., Elkon, K.B. and Reinitz, E. (1985). Lupus pregnancy. II. Unusual pattern of hypocomplementemia and thrombocytopenia in the pregnant patient. *Arthritis Rheum.*, **28,** 58–66
32. Balow, J.E., Austin, H.A., Muenz, L.R., Joyce, K.M., Antonovych, T.T., Klippel, J.H., Steinberg, A.D., Plutz, P.H. and Decker, J.L. (1984). Effect of treatment on the evolution of renal abnormalities in lupus nephritis. *N. Engl. J. Med.*, **311,** 491–495
33. Dinant, H.J., Decker, J.L., Klippel, J.H., Balow, J.E., Plotz, P.H. and Steinberg, A.D. (1982). Alternative modes of cyclophosphamide and azathioprine therapy in lupus nephritis. *Ann. Intern. Med.*, **96,** 728–736
34. Carette, S., Klippel, J.H., Decker, J.W., Austin, H.A., Plotz, P.H., Steinberg, A.D. and Balow, J.E. (1983). Controlled studies of oral immunosuppressive drugs in lupus nephritis: a long-term follow-up. *Ann. Intern. Med.*, **99,** 1–8
35. Donadio, J.V., Halley, K.E., Waganer, R.D., Ferguson, R.H. and McDuffie, F.C. (1974). Further observations on the treatment of lupus nephritis with prednisone and combined prednisone and azathioprine. *Arthritis Rheum.*, **17,** 573–581
36. Fraser, F.C. and Fainstat, T.D. (1951). Production of congenital defects in the offspring of pregnant mice treated with cortisone: progress report. *Pediatrics*, **8,** 527–533
37. Kalter, H. and Warkany, J. (1959). Experimental production of congenital abnormalities in mammals by metabolic procedure. *Physiol. Rev.*, **39,** 69–115
38. Bangiovanni, A.M. and McPadden, A.J. (1960). Steroids during pregnancy and possible fetal consequences. *Fertil. Steril.*, **11,** 181–186
39. European Dialysis and Transplant Association Registration Committee (1987). Combined reports on regular dialysis and transplantation in Europe, *XVII*, 1986. Presented at the *XXIVth Congress of the European Dialysis and Transplant Association – European Renal Association*, October 25–29, Berlin (West)
40. Merrill, J.A. (1955). Cortisone in disseminated lupus erythematosus during pregnancy. Report of a case and review of the literature. *Obstet. Gynecol.*, **6,** 637–643
41. Oppenheimer, E.H. (1964). Lesions in the adrenals of an infantl1 following corticosteroid therapy. *Bull. Johns Hopkins Hosp.*, **114,** 146–151
42. Hodgman, J.E., Elhassani, S. and Dubois, E.L. (1967). Growth and development of children born to steroid treated mothers. Presented at the *Western Society for Pediatric Research*, Los Angeles
43. Burkett, G. (1985). Lupus nephropathy and pregnancy. *Clin. Obstet. Gynecol.*, **28,** 310–323
44. Grigor, R.R., Shervington, P.C., Hughes, G.R.V. and Hawkins, D.F. (1977). Outcome of pregnancy in systemic lupus erythematosus. *Proc. R. Soc. Med.*, **70,** 99–100
45. Hayslett, J.P. (1982). Effect of pregnancy in patients with systemic lupus erythematosus. *Am. J. Kidney Dis.*, **2,** (1 suppl. 1), 223–228

46. Greenberg, L.H. and Tanaka, K.R. (1964). Congenital anomalies probably induced by cyclophosphamide. *J. Am. Med. Assoc.* **188,** 423–426
47. Toledo, T.M., Harper, R.C. and Moser, R.H. (1971). Fetal effects during cyclophosphamide and irradiation therapy. *Ann. Intern. Med.*, **74,** 87–91
48. Hubbard, H.C. and Putney, B. (1979). Systemic lupus erythematosus in pregnancy treated with plasmapheresis. *Br. J. Dermatol.*, **101,** 87–89
49. Pritchard M.H , Jessop, J.D., Trenchard P. and Whitaker, J.A. (1978). Systemic lupus erythematosus. Repeated abortions and thrombocytopenia. *Ann. Rheum. Dis.*, **37,** 476–478
50. Naden, R.P. and Redman, C.W.G. (1985). Antihypertensive drugs in pregnancy. *Clin. Perinatol.*, **12,** 521–538
51. Cockburn, J., Moar, V.A., Ounsted, M. and Redman, C.W. (1982). Final report of study on hypertension during pregnancy: the effects of specific treatment on the growth and development of the children. *Lancet*, **1,** 647–649
52. Ounsted, M.K., Moar, V.A., Good, F.J. and Redman, C.W. (1980). Hypertension during pregnancy with and without specific treatment: the children at the age of 4 years. *Br. J. Obstet. Gynaecol.*, **87,** 19–24
53. Gant, N.F., Madden, J.D., Siiteri, P.K. and MacDonald, P.C. (1976). The metabolic clearance rate of dehydroisoandrosterone sulphate IV: active effects of induced hypertension, hypertension and naturesis in normal and hypertensive pregnancies. *Am. J. Obstet. Gynecol.*, **124,** 143–148
54. Mitra, S., Vertes, V., Roza, O. and Berman, L.B. (1970). Periodic haemodialysis in pregnancy. *Am. J. Med. Sci.*, **259,** 333–339
55. Gimovsky, M.L., Benner, P., Montoro, M., Matt, L.D., Berne, T. and Paul, R. (1983). Successful pregnancy in a patient with systemic lupus erythematosus, renal transplantation and chronic renal failure. *J. Reprod. Med.*, **28,** 677–680
56. Mor-Joseph, S., Navot, D., Rabinovitz, R. and Schenker, J.G. (1984). Collagen disease in pregnancy. *Obstet. Gynecol. Surv.*, **39,** 67–83
57. Davison, J.M., Katz, A.I. and Lindheimer, M.D. (1985). Kidney disease and pregnancy: obstetric outcome and long term renal prognosis. *Clin. Perinatol.*, **12,** 497–519
58. Magey, D.A., Fortner, K.J. and Linder, J. (1983). Pregnancy complicated by periarteritis nodosa: induced abortion as an alternative. *Am. J. Obstet. Gynecol.*, **147,** 103–105
59. Spellacy, W.N. and Janda, G.W. (1964). Scleroderma and pregnancy. *Obstet. Gynecol.*, **23,** 297–300
60. Slate, W.G. and Graham, A.R. (1968). Scleroderma and pregnancy. *Am. J. Obstet. Gynecol.*, **101,** 335–341
61. Knupp, M.Z. and O'Leary, J.A. (1971). Pregnancy and scleroderma, systemic sclerosis. *J. Fla. Med. Assoc.*, **58,** 28–30

INDEX

GPSR Compliance

The European Union's (EU) General Product Safety Regulation (GPSR) is a set of rules that requires consumer products to be safe and our obligations to ensure this.

If you have any concerns about our products, you can contact us on ProductSafety@springernature.com

In case Publisher is established outside the EU, the EU authorized representative is:

Springer Nature Customer Service Center GmbH
Europaplatz 3
69115 Heidelberg, Germany

Batch number: 10761599

Printed by Printforce, the Netherlands